Creating and Marketing Your Birth-Related Business

A Practical Guide

Second Edition

Connie L. Livingston

and

Heather M. Livingston

Foreword by Harriette Hartigan

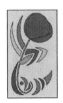

Praeclarus Press, LLC

www.PraeclarusPress.com

Praeclarus Press, LLC

2504 Sweetgum Lane

Amarillo, Texas 79124 USA

806-367-9950

www.PraeclarusPress.com

DISCLAIMER

The information contained in this publication is advisory only and
is not intended to replace sound clinical judgments or individu-
alized patient care. The author disclaims all warranties, whether
expressed or implied, including any warranty as the quality, ac-
curacy, safety, or suitability of this information for any particular
purpose.

ISBN: 9781939807410

Cover Design: Ken Tackett

Acquisition & Development: Kathleen Kendall-Tackett

Copy Editing: Chris Tackett

Layout & Design: Todd Rollison

Operations: Scott Sherwood

To my loving husband Jim, who stands by my side always, and to my amazing daughters, Heather and Erin, whose births inspire me daily.

— Connie

To Mom, the greatest co-author a daughter could have;

To Dad, who always inspires me to do my very best;

To Erin, my sister, best friend, confidant, and cause of endless smiles;

To Erika, who spent endless nights with me in grad school business classes, knowing that one day, we would accomplish great things.

Here is one of my great things.

—Heather

Table of Contents

Foreword

Creating and Marketing Your Birth-Related Business is an excellent and valuable guide for those who want to reach potential clients and customers with their services and products.

Connie Livingston is a childbirth educator, birth advocate, and businesswoman. Livingston synthesizes her experience and expertise with clear and accurate information, encouraging readers to learn and to use the dynamic benefits of business planning, marketing, advertising, and social media.

Midwives, doulas, educators, lactation consultants, and birth artists; this book is for you! *Creating and Marketing Your Birth-Related Business* gives a practical sense of possibilities and concise strategies for birthing and nurturing an effective business, to achieve your mission and goals.

—Harriette Hartigan
Midwife, researcher, and photographer
InSight Photography
www.harriettehartigan.com

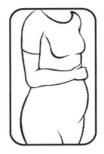

From the Authors

Connie L. Livingston

A Journey

From my very first experience with birthing women while in nursing school in the 1970s, to my childbirth education clients and doula clients in 2015, I continue to be passionate about this business of birth. Through the natural childbirth movement of the 70s, co-optation of childbirth education by hospitals in the 80s, the rise of epidurals in the 90s, and the renewal of the natural childbirth movement in the 2000s, women do not change. How we care for women can change. We can care about how we care for women. If necessary, we can change how we care for women.

A Passion

Some who know me would call it a vocation—or *obsession*. I am passionate about women obtaining accurate information about perinatal health. In today's environment, however, some women are not being told the truth. It is extremely clear that many maternity-care providers are not practicing evidence-based care; they are practicing care as they learned it to be how many years ago. Some are practicing convenient care. Some are practicing care to only avoid litigation.

A Duty

It is our duty as educators, doulas, and consultants in this field to honor the process of childbirth as a woman passes into motherhood. It is our duty to preserve the reverence. It is our duty to remind generation after generation that while technology is good, and we often need it, what has been tried and true for centuries--the gentle way of birthing—is the best option most of the time.

On our *journey* with our *passion* to fulfill our *duty*, we must not forget that we are the keepers of the sacred space. We are the wise women, or *sage femmes*, that will pass down to the generations the preciousness of normal birth.

This book is dedicated to establishing the foundation of business, and the art of passing down of information. Today, sharing information does not only happen person-to-person. Rather, it is also shared on websites, blogs, Facebook, Twitter, and other social media. To meet the needs of the Gen X and Gen Y learners today, social media is a necessary part of any business strategy.

Heather M. Livingston

To have a passion is a great thing. To be able to channel that passion to help others is an even greater thing.

This book is a road map—you already know where you want to go. You know you want to create your own business, and help mothers, fathers, and other educators. Or maybe you're hesitating because starting your own business seems like the most difficult and complex thing to do. A risk. But the greatest risk is risking nothing—especially when you have something you are passionate about. Having the freedom to be your most creative, to work for yourself, make your own decisions, and hold yourself to the highest standards that you set so that you can live out your vision, well, there is nothing like it.

You can reach your goals in many different ways, and you'll have to decide what is right for you, depending on your type of business and your work style. But if you have the passion, and you're ready for the journey, I want this book to be your guide. So, let's get started, because I can't wait to travel with you on your greatest adventure!

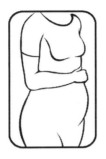

Chapter 1

The Business Side of Birth: Getting Started

Birth is not only about making babies. Birth is about making mothers—strong, competent, capable mothers who trust themselves and know their inner strength.

—Barbara Katz Rothman

Barbara Katz Rothman could have easily been talking about the birth entrepreneur when she made the statement about "trust[ing] themselves and know[ing] their inner strength." While it may sound romantic to be a small, woman-owned business, it is also a lot of hard work from the very beginning!

When Perinatal Education Associates, Inc. was founded in 1999, it started with a home computer and $500. Today, Perinatal Education Associates, Inc. has two websites (www.birthsource.com and www.the-birthfacts.com), a blog (www.childbirthtoday.blog-spot.com), a Facebook page (www.facebook.com/Birthsource), three books, an educational division, and ships products from the online store worldwide. None of this would have been possible without trust and in-ner-strength--and some business smarts.

Another necessity in starting your own business is support: emotional and physical support from fami-ly members. Your business may require long hours and trips out of town to teach workshops and class-es, work with clients, or exhibit at conferences. This type of commitment is only possible with support from family. Family members need to realize that this is a business: a real job with real commitments. If the family assumes that this is "Mom's hobby," then Mom will never become the business woman she aspires to be. It is also, in the beginning, a full-time job. There is paperwork with deadlines and appointments need to be kept. If your family realizes that this is your job and not a hobby, congratulations! You have reached a goal that, unfortunately, many woman who own business-es do not achieve.

Small-Business Fundamentals

Each individual business will be unique. However, there are basics that are common to beginning any small business. Here are seven steps to creating your business.

Step 1: Develop Your Business Plan

A business plan is a written description of your birth-related business, which can change over time. However, it is critical for you to think about all the aspects of your business before you dive in. Should you ever need financial assistance, either through a bank loan or investors, the first thing they will request to see is your business plan.

If your product/service was a party, your business plan is the invitation, but in much greater detail. It is a glimpse of what your business is all about: the *who, what, when, where, and why*. The plan should include details on a variety of all-encompassing areas including the business environment, description of products or services you will offer, a marketing plan, an operation plan, a financial plan, and a financial proposal, if necessary. See Chapter 2 for an in-depth look at writing your business plan.

Step 2: Determining the Legal Structure

Once you have a plan, you must determine what type of business best suits your needs. There are several types of businesses to consider: *sole proprietorship, a partnership, a limited liability company (LLC) and a corporation.*

• A *sole-proprietorship* is a form of business in which one person owns all the assets of the business, and is personally liable for the business. This is the simplest to form and income is reported on your personal taxes. The drawback to this form is that your personal property may be in jeopardy should litigation be brought against you.

• A *partnership* is a type of business comprised of one or more general partners who manage the business and who are personally liable for the partnership debts. This is also relatively simple to form and works well when a clear division of duties and responsibilities is established. The drawbacks of this form are that the partners are personally liable for each other's debts, as if you were married, and your personal property could be in jeopardy by litigation.

• A *limited liability company* is a form of business organization that is managed by its members or managers, characterized by limited liability, and has limitations on the transferability of ownership interest. The forms for a limited liability company are not very difficult to file, as the owners are not personally liable for company matters, and they are not double-taxed.

- *A corporation-subchapter S or subchapter C* can be formed. A subchapter S is designed for small businesses with no more than 35 shareholders. Income is reported on personal income tax forms and there is protection from liability. The subchapter C is for large businesses with unlimited shareholders and investors and double taxation. For corporations, a large drawback is the lengthy paperwork required for filing.

If you live in the U.S., you can get more information on choosing the right type of business for you from the Small Business Administration, Internal Revenue Service (IRS), and the Secretary of State Office of your state.

Step 3: Filing the Proper Forms

It is vital to file the proper tax forms with the federal, state, and local government to ensure that your business stays legal. When you form a business, you are typically advised as to the forms you will need to complete. It is essential that you file the forms on time so as to not incur additional fees. Figure A is a chart of the typical tax forms you will need to file based on your type of business. Additional forms to record your business income will need to be filed with your county and state governments, so check with your Secretary of State Office, your county Auditor, and the IRS to make certain you file all the forms you need.

	Individual Taxes	You may be liable for	Use Form
Sole Proprietor		Income tax	1040 and Schedule C or C-EZ
		Self-employment tax	1040 and Schedule SE
		Estimated tax	1040-ES
Sole Proprietor	Yes	Social Security and Medicare taxes and income tax withholding	944
	Yes	Federal Unem-ployment (FUTA) tax	940
Partnership		Annual return of income for busi-ness	1065
		Employment taxes	Same as sole proprietor
Partners	Yes	Income tax	1040 and Form 1120
	Yes	Self-employment tax	1040 and C-EZ if reporting less than $5000
	Yes	Estimated tax	1040
Corporation or S Corp.		Income tax	11205 1120 Sch. K-1
		Estimated	1120-W
		Employment taxes	940 & 941
S Corp shareholders	Yes	Income tax	1040 and Schedule E
	Yes	Estimated tax	1040ES

Figure A. Business Forms Required by Company Type.

Source: www.irs.gov accessed 3/1/2015

Step 4: Organization is the Key

Once you have developed your business plan, chosen the type of business that best suits your needs, and filed the proper forms to make it all legal, you'll want to work on organizing the business.

Finance Management

By now, you should already have established a bank account separate from your personal account. This is the first step in establishing credit for your business. It can be your avenue to also apply for a business credit card if you so choose. Remember, as with personal credit cards, it is best to pay off all debts each month rather than carry any balance and accumulate interest.

As you organize your business, be sure to inquire about the use of other professionals, such as an attorney, a website designer, an accountant, etc., who can aid you in starting your business. You will also need to determine what type of office equipment you may need. Most will need, at the minimum, a computer, printer, work area, filing cabinet (or other filing system), Internet access, and a specific email account. You may even choose to have a separate business phone line.

With regards to software for your computer, it is a good idea to purchase an accounting software program, such as *Quick Books Pro*, to aid with all the accounting issues. Many accounting software programs will interface with tax programs. For example, for S Corporations, TurboTax for Business interfaces with Quick Books. You will be able to keep track of all your account balances, sales, accounts receivables, accounts payables, tax information, employee pay, budgets, balance sheets, etc. A program such as this also creates personal, professional invoices for your clients.

Refer to the end of this chapter and the worksheet with two columns: one side is "Necessary" and the other is "Nice." Write down all of the things that you need to purchase to start your business. As you write these things down, be honest with yourself in knowing how much start-up funding you have. Maybe you won't be able to purchase everything in your "Nice" list now, but these items can be on your list of goals and rewards to yourself and your business as you grow. Maybe you start with your home desktop computer to get yourself going, but after six months of sales, you can afford a laptop.

After you've made a list of the things you need to buy, write down all of your costs. There are essentially two types of costs: *fixed costs* and *variable costs*. Fixed costs are things that are a certain amount that you have to pay at regular intervals. One example could be your phone bill. You know that you have to pay $40 every month for your cell phone service.

Variable costs are things that vary depending on how much you sell. For example, let's say that you are a prenatal massage therapist. Perhaps your one-hour massage service includes fresh linens on your massage table or (scented/non-scented) massage oil. How much are your variable costs for selling that one massage?

Massage Variable Costs

Launder Linens	$5.00
Massage Oil	$40.00 (gallon)
Diffuser	$20.00**
Total:	$65.00+

One time purchase, amortized over several massages.

So, for every massage you sell, it costs you $65.00. This doesn't include how much your time and expertise is worth. You may also have one-time costs. In this case, perhaps it's your phone you use to talk with clients. A phone should last you a while, and while the usage of the phone will eventually lead to it needing to be replaced, that replacement is unforeseeable and not a cost you have to think about every month. It is something to plan for as you think about saving your profits.

Now, as you think about your costs or expenses to make your business run, you can connect this to the price of your product or service. Let's go back to the massage example. For simplicity's sake, let's say that your massage business advertises in the local newspaper, you purchase a phone for clients to call you and to set up appointments, you have a monthly phone bill, and you have the above variable costs. Your budget would look like this:

Prenatal Massage Business Budget

Fixed Costs (monthly)

Phone bill	$40.00
Local Health Magazine Ad	$50.00
Space for Service (Rent)	$200+
Launder linens per massage	
Massage oil	$40.00
Cell phone	$40.00

One-Time Costs

Diffuser	$20.00

So, if you only sell one massage in one month, it costs you $390. If you sold your massage for that amount, you'd break even. If you want to make a profit, you'll need to factor in an additional amount to add to the price. If you decide to charge $60 for a one-hour massage and do two massages, you cannot make a profit. If you sell seven massages in one month at $60 each, you will make a total profit of $30.00. Here is the math:

# of items/services sold X price = Sales

Sales - fixed costs – one-time costs – (variable costs X # of items sold) = Total Profit

Total Profit / # of items sold = profit per each item sold

This can become complicated the more costs and elements you add. There are college courses on business budgeting and accounting. The main points to consider are:

1. What are all the costs of running your business?

2. Given all your costs, what price should you charge so that you make a profit?

3. How much profit do you want or need to make?

Once you have your profit, think about how to spend that money: buy inventory/supplies, attend continuing education offerings or conferences, purchase more equipment, spend more on advertising, save for a bigger purchase, invest and use the interest from the investment, or maybe a combination!

While not legally required for tax purposes, having a separate bank account for your business is important because you should not mix your *business* and *personal* money. Having a bank account in your business's name is the way to go. As mentioned previously, you may also want to invest in a professional finance software program, such as Quick Books Pro, to keep track of your business finances. At tax time, simply hand a copy of last year's activity to your accountant.

Separate Space for your Office

A separate room for your office would be nice, but it is not mandatory. But you do need an area that is distinctly your workspace with the look and feel of your birthing personality. Perhaps it has photos or illustrations that inspire you. Newspaper clippings or even sculptures of pregnant women? Birth photos or a Rebozo hanging; all of this helps you to transition from your personal life to your professional life when all of your lives are under the same roof. Ideally, the space can be closed off from the rest of the house by partitions, dividers, drapes, or even a shower curtain, if that is all you have. Often, because we have a difficult time placing importance on this work, it's important not to use your dining room table as a desk. You will either have no place to eat or have all of your "sorted" paperwork resorted each time there is a meal.

Separate Phone and Internet Connection

Your clients will appreciate their calls being answered by you, your assistant, or a professional-sounding voicemail message. A separate phone line for your business might be helpful so that you can "quit" for the day. Consider the cost of adding a second line to your existing cell phone account. For internet access, see if your cell phone carrier can supply you with an internet card which can be plugged into a USB port in your computer or you can use your phone as a "hot spot." Then the cost for the access can be bundled onto your cell phone bill. Fax machines are no longer a necessity in business—simply tell a customer you have "gone green" and send them a bill or sales receipt as a PDF (portable document format) via email. However, if they must send a fax, you may want to investigate a free fax service, such as efax.com, or if your local UPS or FedEx Stores have a fax service.

Website and Email Account in your Business Name

For the "birth junkie," much can be learned on the web. For mothers with young children, the web is easily accessed 24 hours a day (regardless of time zones) and contains the most up-to-date information from around the world. Web-active birth professionals get 75% to 90% of their clients from the Internet via organizational membership sites, free referral sites, or social media.

Consider a website for business and marketing purposes. It helps people to know your philosophy, get a feel for the type of person you are, and appeals to those who are internet savvy. Be sure to have reciprocal links with affiliating organizations. More tips on websites and the Internet are in Chapters 4 and 5.

Business License and Federal Tax ID Number

Your city or county may require you to have a business license; it varies per jurisdiction. Contact your local governments to find out, especially your Secretary of State website. If getting a tax identification number is a must, obtain this number from the Internal Revenue Service (IRS). Should you want to sell products made by other people, you'll need your tax identification number to prove you are a reseller so you can get these products at wholesale prices. Additionally, if you sell, for example, birth balls to hospitals, they will need a W9 form with your business name, address, and tax identification number to prove credibility. To make copies of W9s, you can visit the IRS website for a fillable form, and then sign and date as necessary.

Insurance

Many birth professionals state that since childbirth educators, doulas, or lactation educators do no clinical tasks, or perform no medical procedures, it is unlikely that they will be sued. That being said, in our litigious society, anyone and everyone can be named in a lawsuit. If your business is incorporated and you are sued, the only thing they can take from you is the money in your business account. If you are not incorporated, then your house, car and belongings are at risk. There are several insurance companies that do provide liability or malpractice insurance, so take the time to investigate this thoroughly.

If you are working out of your home, check with your homeowners' insurance company about supplying you or your business with fire and theft insurance for inventory, small business insurance, or partnership insurance (protects you from lawsuits arising from the actions or omissions by any of your business partners). If you are not working out of your home, consider applying for these types of insurances, plus general liability insurance. General liability insurance covers negligence resulting in injury when clients are in your office area.

> *"Create your own referral network. Team up with other professionals to offer discounts or extras (i.e., free prenatal yoga class at [insert name] studio with a prenatal massage)."*
>
> *~Kathi Kizirnis*
> *Co-director of*
> *Practice Yoga on*
> *Fifth*

Regular Business Hours, and a Life Outside Your Office

Experienced home-based business women say they set regular business hours and stick to them. For many independents, starting a home-based business means blurring the lines between work and family life. Find the happy medium between working on your laptop with the baby nursing, and isolating yourself from family and friends. When it is not business hours, let your business voicemail get the call. Close the door on the office.

Step 5: Creating a Professional Image

The Name of Your Business

Decide on the name of your business and image you wish to portray. Who is your intended target de-mographic and what would appeal to them? Do you want a logo that is cute or sweet (e.g., a cartoon of a baby, baby blocks, stork, etc.), symbolic in nature (e.g., symbol of pregnant belly, mother and child, ancient symbols), or a logo based on the name of your company? Names and logos will be discussed in a later chapter.

What You Produce Reflects on You

Create your business cards and brochures, making them clear, concise, eye-catching, and informative. Do not put too much or too little information on the card or brochure. Gather cards and brochures from others in the field to collect ideas for your own. Even though you can give a great first impression with the marketing materials you create, in order to maintain that favorable impression, remember to dress and act the part as well.

General Professionalism

The old adage is true: first impressions *do* matter. Dress and act in keeping with the type of audience you will be addressing, whether it is a professional group of physicians and hospital personnel or a group of pregnant teens. What you wear can say a lot about you. It is important to still value your individuality while giving a professional appearance that adds to your credibility as a professional.

Also consider how you allow electronic media to present you. Clients will make judgments about you and you aren't even there! Consider your voicemail message, ring back tones, and email signature. Are they clear and professional? While "Hey, you know what to do!" may be perfectly acceptable for your personal voicemail, you may want to consider something more professional for your business line. Also, think about social media and how you are represented in the photos you post. A picture is worth a thousand words, whether they are true or just inferences.

Step 6: Advertise Your Services

The best advertising may be the least expensive. Advertising your services on websites can be very effective and is, oftentimes, free. You can also get your local newspaper to write a story on the newest business in town; yours! Attending conferences, workshops, and other professional events affords you the opportunity to network with others who could send clients your way. Find opportunities to talk about your services to the general public through presentations or exhibits at baby fairs, bookstores, community centers, clinics, and more. Think of all the places you will find your clientele and organize ways to get the word of your business to them. Creativity breeds success. Never stop selling your services!

I get my clients' provider's names and addresses. I send a letter to them introducing myself, letting them know that I have been hired by a mutual client, that I look forward to working with them (the doctor or midwife), and hope to complement their care. I also do a letter after the delivery stating that I enjoyed working alongside them, and telling them what a wonderful experience it was (if it was indeed a wonderful one!!!), and hope to be able to work with them again in the future. I put in the letter if they think I could be of assistance to any of their other patients to feel free to give out my information. I will then call the office a few days later and speak with the office manager, and let them know I did a delivery with "Dr. So and So," and was wondering if I may be able to put some of my contact information in their office. Most have said yes!!!

Dona Grassity CD (DONA), CIMI, Joliet, IL
Special Delivery Doula Service & More

Step 7: Self-Evaluation

Periodically, it is necessary to examine what works, what doesn't, what areas are weak, and what is strong. Keep a chart on your marketing efforts and how those efforts pay off. Perhaps you decide to use a code in your online store to track the types of discounts you offer (e.g., you use the word "doula" to track discounted sales for International Doula Month in May or gift sales in December using the word "Holiday"). Perhaps you have a special offer for your followers on Facebook or Twitter. Sales may increase substantially by using a social media mini-campaign.

When speaking with clients or customers on the phone, ask how they heard about your services. Perhaps it was a well-placed brochure, business card, or even a direct-mail postcard. Receiving this type of feedback can tell you what is working and what is not.

Words of Wisdom: An Interview with Michelle Hardy

Michelle Hardy is a birth entrepreneur from Milwaukee, Wisconsin. Michelle had a vision to form a non-profit organization to serve women based on their ability to pay. She began working on the idea in late 2010.

By 2011, "Mothering the Mother" became a non-profit corporation. "We didn't have our first brick and mortar until 2013," says Michelle. "Prior to that, we used rooms in churches, high schools, and libraries where we could meet with clients or teach classes."

What is Michelle's most powerful marketing tool?

It is definitely word of mouth. We have some printed material. And in the beginning, quite literally, I would go online to search for local obstetricians to obtain their addresses and phone numbers. I then called them to set up an appointment to see them. Some consented and some did not. Regardless, I sent our information every 6 months. Soon, I began to see referrals.

Michelle said that the logo for Mothering the Mother, Inc. was created by her then 15- year-old daughter, noting "teens can be unbelievably creative and insightful." She then enlisted the help of a local college student majoring in graphics to refine the logo.

With the help of GoDaddy for hosting, Michelle maintains the Mothering the Mother's website. Laughing that she learned HTML coding in the early days of the web, Michelle is now happy for programs that work like Microsoft Word, and for free forms designs, such as jotform.com.

What tips would Michelle give for those just beginning a business?

Be persistent. When you initially create print advertising, money going out. I would take our print advertising and give presentations to midwives, WIC, and Health Depts. Truthfully, some were nervous and hesitant that we would steal their clients. We reassured them that we offered complementary programs and we were not competitors.

We also demonstrated what set us apart. We defined what a "good" doula was by referencing our scope of practice. Several providers had somewhat negative experiences with doulas who chose to practice outside of their scope.

In the birth world, one big mistake is to go superfast and expect finding clients and getting income to be super easy. The reality is that referrals take at least 2 years.

WorkSheet I

The Birth Biz
Self-Assessment

Potential name of your business:

_____

Having a successful birth-related business means:

_____

_____

_____

_____

_____

_____

_____

_____

_____

The initial obstacles to your business are:

_____

_____

_____

_____

_____

_____

_____

_____

_____

_____

List some of your personal strengths:

_____

_____

_____

_____

_____

_____

_____

_____

_____

_____

List some of your personal weaknesses:

_____

_____

_____

_____

_____

_____

_____

_____

_____

_____

What kind of support will you need as you start your business?

_____

_____

_____

_____

_____

_____

_____

_____

_____

_____

As your business grows, what other type of support will you need?

_____

_____

_____

_____

_____

_____

_____

_____

_____

_____

What are your short-term goals?

_____

_____

_____

_____

_____

_____

_____

_____

_____

_____

What are your long-term goals?

_____

_____

_____

_____

_____

_____

_____

_____

_____

_____

_____

_____

How will your business benefit the birthing business?

_____

_____

_____

_____

_____

_____

_____

_____

_____

_____

What will be the legal structure of your company?

- Sole proprietor
- Partnership
- Limited Liability (LLC)
- Corporation (Corp)

Go to the Secretary of State's website for your state and then list the forms (tax and otherwise) you will need to become a legal entity in your state:

_____

_____

_____

_____

List some of the start-up items you will need for your business:

*Nice*_____

_____

_____

_____

_____

_____

_____

_____

_____

*Necessary*_____

_____

_____

_____

_____

_____

_____

_____

_____

_____

_____

What are your fixed costs? One-time costs? Variable costs?

_____

_____

_____

_____

_____

_____

_____

_____

_____

_____

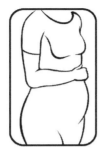

Chapter 2

Your Business Plan

Whenever you offer new ideas or approaches, you have to expect resistance and allow time for change. I have found being consistent and persistent with offerings has helped bring our "new idea" more into the mainstream. Set goals, intentions and always reevaluate where you are. Know that planting seeds is just the beginning process; you must always remember to water and fertilize these seeds regularly with love and your vision.

— Jennifer Shryock
Owner, Family Paws

As you stand at the base of "Starting My Own Business" mountain, it may seem like it is an impossible mountain to climb, so here are seven elements for creating your business plan:

I.   Executive Summary

The executive summary is a one-to-two page description of your business. You should also include a Mission Statement. Why should you create a mission statement? It is the very heart of your business; your calling card that defines the business and its main objectives. Your mission statement helps you to keep steadfast to your original goals and ideals. As you grow, it is the checks and balances in decision making. Asking yourself, "Is this choice in line with my mission statement?" will help your business to be focused on what is really important to you and what your business is founded upon. There are three components to a mission statement:

A. Customer needs, or *what* is being satisfied

B. Customer groups, or *who* is being satisfied

C. The businesses activities or competencies, or how the needs are being satisfied.

You can research any company, organization, university, or hospital and find their mission statement as an example. While yours shouldn't be an exact copy, seeing how others word their mission statement can give you some ideas or inspire you as you formulate yours. Here are a couple of examples:

> *As a childbirth educator, I provide childbirth classes to expectant teens. My classes are focused on easing the anxiety and tension by using a specially designed curriculum geared towards teenagers with in-depth explanations and simplistic diagrams, as well as optional pairing with volunteer doula services.*

> *Lactation Ladies, Inc. is a team of skilled lactation consultants who assist mothers who are learning to breastfeed their first child. By offering a wide variety of lactation equipment, as well as in-home instruction, Lactation Ladies, Inc. is a personalized service for the woman wanting help with something so personal.*

Explain in a few paragraphs your short-term (12 to 18 months) and long-term (2 to 5 years) goals for the company. How fast do you think it will grow? The executive summary introduces your business strategy. These goals and objectives help to keep you focused, especially under times of stress. Don't be afraid to dream. That is how great things are accomplished. Dream big!

II. History and Overview

History and Overview includes the purpose of the company or why you created the business: the business history—the history of the creation; benefits—how will your company benefit the birthing business and how is it unique; the goals of your business (think about your mission statement); and critical success factors--what will you measure your success by? Number of services or products sold, estimated financial growth, and number of partners, associates, or employees.

Since this section gives a brief overview of the business and the history behind it, it can be a timeline of development formatted in text. You can discuss your background, education, experiences, and skills that have led you into the creation of the business and discussion of the recent history of the company, its products and services, staffing etc. Writing this section gives you a historic look at where you've been and what initiatives have been established during the last few years. Some examples of major events would include the hiring of a sales staff, achieving any certifications or awards, major increase in marketing budget, major new product introductions, newly established joint ventures, creation of company website, etc.

In the birth profession, many find this section helpful on those days when we question our passion and beliefs. The birth profession basically has two tracks of thought: the Medical Model of Care, and the Holistic/Midwifery Model of Care. The chart listing Holistic-Model Beliefs and Medical-Model Beliefs can help to identify where a business lies.

Holistic-Model Beliefs	Medical-Model Beliefs
Birth is a natural and normal process	Birth is a crisis that needs to be managed for safety
Medications and machines are tools that are there if the need arises	Medications and machines are a vital part of all births
There are instinctual and emotional components to labor and birth and they both impact the process	Labor is a physical process that can be managed with medication and interventions
There are spiritual and sexual components to the labor and birth process	Spirituality and sexuality of birth is rarely acknowledged
Pregnancy and birth are experiences of health	Pregnancy and birth are hazardous times for a woman and she is in need of a medical rescue
A woman's body knows how to birth. She is in control	Medical staff is necessary for a positive pregnancy outcome. Staff are in control
Empowered women have emotional and physical support, use comfort measures and may only need slight medication for birth	Natural childbirth (without any medication) is barbaric. Analgesia and anesthesia are necessary for birth
There is beauty and power in the birthing process and bringing life into the world	Much can go wrong and it's important to avoid distress at all costs
Birth is a rite of passage that profoundly touches a woman's heart and soul for the rest of her life	Birth happens. It is simply a few hours out of a woman's life

Chances are, your business will land in the Holistic Model. Regardless, it is important for you to achieve self-awareness about you and your business's philosophy on the work. If you are not firm in your philosophical underpinnings, it will be difficult to brand and sell your services/products to others.

III. Business Environment

We are challenged in the birth business. As business owners, we need to see our fellow birth professionals not only as colleagues with whom to refer, work with, and network, but also as the competition.

Creating your business is, in the rawest of terms, an invasion into the birth industry. You need to scout out the lay of the land, so that you know what you are up against before you begin your campaign. In World War II, General Patton knew that a tank battle was eminent with his adversary General Rommel, who considered himself such an expert in tank warfare that he wrote an extensive book describing his perfected techniques. Patton picked up a copy and read the memoir, all the while devising his strategy, knowing that of his opponent. As Patton defeated Rommel, he exclaimed, "Rommel. I read your book!"

Although we are not at war, the same basic idea applies here. You should know what you are up against in the market. Think about what legal constraints you have. Perhaps you need a certain type of certification to provide a service. Is the market lean or saturated with businesses similar to yours? What is the demand? How many babies are born in your community each year? What share can you expect to have of that number?

If you've ever studied basic economics, you've certainly come across the concept of *supply and demand*. For example, you will be in greater demand if you are in an area where there is little access to childbirth than if you are in an area where there are multiple educators and convenient access to classes. If your area has many options, how would you distinguish your business from others? What makes you stand out? What can you offer clients that no one else can? On the flip side, if you live in an area with little supply of childbirth classes and a great demand, you will need to figure out how you will handle so many requests for childbirth classes!

> *Having a deep passion for the work we do is absolutely essential. But it won't necessarily make you successful in the larger world. To succeed, you need the marriage of a passionate heart and a practical business head.*
>
> *~April Kline*
> *Founder of Dar a Luz Network, Inc.*

You'll also want to think about any problems or hindrances you will have. Detailed analysis of competitors, including strengths and weaknesses, is important, although we do not often like to think of our colleagues as the competition! This section should include an overall competitive analysis: "How do you stack up," as well as complete profiles of your top five competitors. You should try to assess market share of your own company as well as the competition. Identifying them early on will help you figure out the steps to finding solutions.

IV. Description of Product or Service

This is the section where your business takes the spotlight. What makes your product or services the best? What makes your business so unique? What are the features and benefits to what you "sell?"

It is indeed difficult for many in the birthing business to point out their strengths. We tend to be helpers and pleasers, somewhat timid and shy when it comes to drawing comparisons to others. However, it is time to throw timid out the door and just be honest. What features do you have that others don't? Features vs. benefits can sometimes be used interchangeably, but they are different. A *feature* is an attribute, and a *benefit* is what a feature does for the customer. For example, a feature of a DVD is that it has a scene selection op-tion in the Menu. The benefit of a DVD is that you can avoid fast forwarding and choose a desired spot in the DVD using the scene selection feature. Identifying the features and benefits helps you to distinguish how your product or service differs from others. This will be helpful as you look at product/service differentia-tion in your marketing. You will also want to discuss whether you own any legal rights to a product/service such as a patent or license, as well as how you produce the product

V. Marketing Plan

Marketing is a process by which, in this case, birth professionals find out what the consumers want both in terms of services and products, and to show the consumers what they want. Marketing is sometimes the most important aspect of business growth. If your customers do not know you exist (lack of consumer awareness), your business will not prosper in the long term. As you first begin to think about your business, consider the 4 P's of Marketing:

Product

What are the actual goods or services that you will provide? Do you offer birth doula care, pregnancy massage, lactation consultation, or belly casting kits for sale? When considering the product, also consider how the pregnant or professional consumer will use this product. If you don't feel that enough consumers will take advantage, consider offering something else that will be more attractive.

Pricing

This refers to the process of setting a price for a product or service. If you are selling a product, generally take the wholesale price for which you have purchased it and double that price for the retail price. However, sometimes it actually pays you to reduce your profit so more people will notice your business by the "good deal" they will be getting by purchasing from you. Services are harder to price, so find out who your competitors are and what they are charging for their services.

Do not short yourself, but be honest. Base the pricing on your years of experience, number of certifications, additional training, and professional background. Think about who your potential customers are. Do they have a lot of options? If you have a lot of competitors, price may be a factor in the customer's decision. What is the socioeconomic status of your clientele? If you work in a poor or lower-middle-class area, you won't want your prices so high that your customers can't afford you. Likewise, you might be able to charge a higher price if you live in an affluent area.

Promotion

This is how you build awareness around your business. It's your advertising and publicity strategy. When developing a budget, especially for a new business, it can be tempting to spend less on advertising, and more in other areas. But be aware, even if you have the best product or service, the best customer service, and highest quality, if no one *knows* about it, they won't buy it! We'll talk more in-depth about advertising, and provide insight and ideas in a later chapter.

Placement

Often called "Place," this refers to how the product or service will get to the consumer. It is often referred to as "distribution." Maybe you will start your business from your home, or maybe you have an office space. Often referred to as "brick and mortar," you will promote your services or products by attracting people to your place of business. If your business is a "dot com" business, you may be completely electronic. Perhaps you have a website with an online store.

Place also refers to how you manage your inventory and process orders. Do you have a separate storage or keep stock on hand? Do you order your stock as the orders come in? There are so many things to consider! If you order inventory as you receive orders, your turnaround time on orders will be long, but you will only have to buy inventory you know will sell. This is called the "just in time" model. You won't have to worry about not selling inventory or inventory getting dust on your shelves.

You may not be eligible for discounts unless you place a larger order. If you purchase inventory and have some in stock, you will need "upfront money" to purchase the inventory that is certain to sell. However, you might increase customer service if you can ship out their order quickly since you already have their items. Remember, you can always do sales or "buy 1, get one ½ off" or other discounts if you are left with inventory that isn't moving off the shelf fast enough.

Many new business owners are apprehensive about taking credit cards, and rely primarily on cash or checks. However, with credit card readers, such as Square, Intuit GoPayment, Payware Mobile, or RO-AMpay, you can attach the readers to your cell phone or mobile device (such as iPad), and make credit card transactions easier. One birth professional noticed a 75% increase in her business when she began taking credit cards. For example, with Square, an average of 2.75% per swipe would deposit $97.25 in your business account (from a $100 transaction) in just one day. You are not limited to the type of card you accept. Square accepts VISA, MasterCard, Discover, and American Express. What about security? Information is encrypted at the moment of swiping, and no information is kept on your phone. The customer signs the image on your device, and a receipt is emailed directly to their inbox.

All of marketing is not the creation of colorful signage, business cards, or flyers/brochures that describe your services/products, although, these are truly vital aspects of marketing. It is also about your demographics and anticipating what the consumer will want in the future, and meeting that need before it actually becomes a need.

Be proactive! To do this, you must have your finger on the pulse of the generation currently birthing! For example, the generation that is birthing TODAY, the Y Generation (often called Millennials), is accustomed to technology, and lots of it. So, childbirth education by PowerPoint, websites, and podcasts are logical next steps in meeting the needs of this generation.

Branding and Marketing

There are two aspects of marketing to consider: branding and advertising. Branding is the aspect of creating memory hooks to associate images, symbols, music, or mottos to immediately identify a product or service. What auto insurance company has a gecko as a spokesperson? What restaurant has the golden arches? What credit card has "what's in YOUR wallet?" as their motto? This is branding.

Advertising is the avenue to promoting the awareness of your brand. It's the communication from you to the customers about three main factors: what the produce/service is, how it benefits the customer/why people should buy it, and how the customer can learn more and purchase it. Although, advertising is such a huge element of your business's success that we've devoted a whole chapter to it, it also warrants a few important points here.

In advertising, photos can speak a thousand words but they can also get you into legal trouble. It's a question of ownership and permission: copyright. Copyright is a form of legal protection for one's ownership over their original works. Stock photos or clipart that comes with computer software are usable, because when you purchase the software, you are paying for the right to use it. A lot of people will go on to the Internet search for a photo, and copy and paste it. This can be really dangerous if you don't have the rights to the photo!

Some photos are free to use and they are marked as such. Others may specifically say that they are copyrighted and that you cannot use them or must contact the owner for permission to use it. Sometimes owners will allow you to use the photo. Other times, they may ask you to give them credit next to the photo. It is a good idea to make sure you receive written permission and keep it on file in case there is ever a dispute about its usage. If there is no note, it is safe to default to the picture being copyrighted.

If you decide to take your own photos, you then own the copyright. However, if you take a photo of someone or their property, they can have rights to the photo as well. It is a best practice to have your model or the owner of the property to sign and date a Photo Release, turning over the ownership of the photo to you. At the end of this chapter, there are samples of language you can use to write your own Photo Release.

Advertising is 25% content, 25% creativity, and 50% psychological. You want people to remember your advertising, and the two senses that greatly assist in this memory recall are visual and auditory. Auditory is more prevalent in radio or TV advertisements. Ever find yourself humming an ad jingle, or are you able to associate a catchy slogan with a business? This is your brain memorizing based on what it is hearing.

Now, to begin your business, you may not be advertising with radio or TV, so using the visual sense will be most important. Two aspects to focus on are advertising colors or images, and organization. The colors you use in your print advertising can denote a feeling or mood just as the words you use. Here are some examples:

Green: Associated with nature; tranquility, good luck, health, jealously, fertility, stress reduction.

Blue: promotes calmness, serenity, can be associated with sadness. It is the leastappetizing color and can lower the pulse rate and body temperature.

Red: Displays love, warmth, comfort, and can be associated with anger, excitement, or intensity.

Yellow: Is cheery and warm. It can fatigue the eye, causing eye strain. It can also create feelings of frustration and increase metabolism. It is one of the most attention-getting colors.

Purple: Symbolizes royalty, wealth, wisdom, and spirituality. It is exotic.

Brown: Symbolizes nature, strength, and reliability. It can create feelings of security, but also sadness. It is also down-to-earth, and conventional.

Orange: Displays energy, excitement, enthusiasm, and warmth. It is used to draw attention.

Pink: Symbolizes love and romance. It is calming. In excessive amounts, it can create

feelings of irritation.

Black: Displays death, mourning, and evil. It also displays a sense of formality or sophistication.

White: Displays purity and innocence. It is cold, bland, and sterile.

Keep in mind that this Color Psychology is influenced by culture. In the United States, black can be associated with death, which is why it's a social norm to wear black to a funeral. In some Asian cultures, however, white is associated with mourning and death.

Images or symbols can also have different meanings as well: making the "OK" symbol with your hands means that everything is okay or good in the U.S. or England. However, in France or Latin America, it is similar to giving someone the middle finger. Depending on where you live, and the demographic in the area of which you are advertising, it is advisable to do some research on those cultures and increase your awareness so you are effective and not accidentally offensive!

Another factor is organization of advertising content. This element is a little more obvious. Essentially, it refers to how you've organized and spaced the content. Is there enough space so that it doesn't seem so full, that you can't easily read it? Are there so many fonts being used that it looks jarring to the eye? Remember to only include the information you must communicate to your customers: the essentials. If you try to include too much information, it could be difficult for the customer to view it and take away the main messages. You are exposed to many ads every day. Think about the ones that you actually pay attention to. Your brain gives something mere seconds to decide whether to move on or take the time to learn more. Your advertising needs to be constructed well, so that the potential customer will take the time to read and possibly further explore what you have to sell.

Look at these simple examples. Which one just looks more appealing?

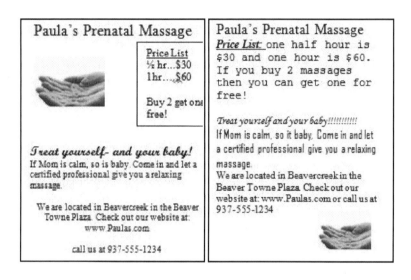

One trick to use if you design the layout is making a few versions. Walk away for about a half-hour, and then come back to all the designs. See which one your eyes are naturally drawn to first. This can be an easy test on which version works best. You can always ask a friend or family member to give you honest feedback!

WorkSheet 2

My Birth Biz Plan

What vision do you have for your business?

_____

_____

_____

_____

_____

_____

_____

_____

Can you put that into a Vision Statement?

_____

_____

_____

_____

_____

_____

_____

What is your Mission Statement?

_____

_____

_____

_____

_____

_____

_____

_____

_____

Will your business be in the Medical Model, Holistic Model, or a blend of both?

_____

_____

_____

_____

_____

_____

_____

_____

_____

Agreement for Photo Release

I _____ (print name) agree that my image may be used for advertising materials for [insert company name].

I understand that I release all rights and privileges to the images. I release the photographer and company form any liability by virtue of any blurring, distortion, alteration, or use in composite form, whether intentional or otherwise, that may occur or be produced in the taking of such photographs or in any subsequent processing of them.

I understand that by signing this release form, I agree to my image's reproduction and that I am not under any obligation to be paid any fees or royalties from its printing and/or usage.

_____   _____

Name   Date

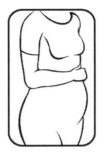

Chapter 3

Overview of Marketing

The point to remember about selling things is that, as well as creating atmosphere and excitement around your products, you've got to know what you're selling.

—Stuart Wilde

As we described in Chapter 1, birth professionals are passionate about their profession and excited about their passion! When setting up your birth-related business, you will have to do more than just be passionate or excited. You will need to put your business hat on for a while and identify your exact target market.

A *target market* is the exact group of individuals you want to reach and who have the greatest potential of purchasing from you. Do you want to serve expectant parents? New parents? Birth professionals? All three?

For many independent childbirth educators and birth professionals, it is difficult to envision what we do as being a real business: a profession. Yet midwives, childbirth educators, antepartum, birth, and postpartum doulas, massage therapists, and lactation consultants or educators ARE business women by definition. We provide a service, and for that service, we are paid by our clients.

Since you are a birth professional, your target market may be expectant women and families. Yet, it is illogical to think that chasing down pregnant women in malls or grocery stores will be profitable. Therefore, subcategories in your target market are the baby fairs and stores where these women visit, and publications that this target market reads. Obtain permission to place your brochure in the offices of physicians/midwives, and perhaps in the offices of the perinatologists who may perform services in your community.

> *It is difficult to look at my doula friend as my back-up and also my competition. I see things in a whole different perspective.*
>
> *~A doula from Utah*

Additionally, hospitals or birthing centers may enjoy handing out brochures during open houses or during tours of their maternity facilities. These brochures may also be placed (again, with permission) in packets at baby fairs, and in maternity or infant stores. Many Babies "R" Us stores have monthly baby fairs and birth professionals find it helpful to participate in these events. If you have extra money for advertising, investigate local parenting publications.

The Market Analysis

A market analysis examines the revenue history and financial forecast for similar businesses. Established businesses can use graphics to chart revenues for the past five years, and project two years into the future. If a business serves both professionals, and expectant and new parents, the chart can be segmented by market niche. This section will give you a good understanding of your company's past performance as it relates to your marketing investments. Also, it should be as detailed as possible because, as you work with the numbers, various strategies will be suggested for the future. For example, you might realize that sales to a particular market are growing at a faster rate than other markets, and yet has received very little marketing investment. Therefore, a strategy might be to increase the marketing investment in this segment.

Marketing Objectives

Within the Market Analysis, you will want to write three or four measurable overall marketing objectives. Usually, it is impossible to accomplish more than three to four major objectives in a given year. It's important to keep your eye on the ball, and these objectives should represent the key objectives for growing your business. They should be easily measurable on a monthly basis, and you should have specific reports (for example, through Quickbooks) that measure each of these objectives. An example would be increasing revenues by 10%.

Following the listing of the marketing objectives should be a discussion of the strategies you will use to achieve those objectives. The difference between an objective and a strategy is that the objective states what you will do and a strategy states how you will do it. Using the example above, there are several strategies which could accomplish the objective of growing revenues by 10%; increase the number of customers, decrease the cost of services/products, enter a new market, or increase the number of catalogs and mailings, etc.

Your mission here is to choose the strategies that fit your company and your services or products. How do you plan to tell the world you are open for business? Will you rely exclusively on word of mouth? Will you advertise in print, television or radio, or on the Web (or all three)?

In order to achieve the marketing objectives, you will need a marketing budget. Will you make brochures or business cards? Where will you place them (Note: Some consider placing brochures or business cards inside of books at bookstores or libraries to be unprofessional)?

The budget, while an uncomfortable topic to many business owners, will help you project both expenses and income. Through mathematics, itemize the estimated income and also the cost of providing your services or products. Include costs of specific marketing channels: direct mail, exhibits, print advertising, business cards, flyers, website, etc. You should analyze results as well.

> *You must hone your vision for your business. And then, every single thing you do must further that vision. That is the only way your message is going to stand out in a saturated field.*
>
> *~Devon Horsman*
> *Founder of Dar a Luz Network, Inc.*

How much business resulted from your investment in print ads? Some channels will be easier to measure than others, but you should try to attribute as much as possible to get a clear picture of how the allocation of your marketing resources affects the ultimate outcome (which is income). Some business owners find that they benefit from creating a chart showing every activity and expense for every month with a total for the year.

As the stock market ebbs and flows, a discussion of current business environment, internal and external issues, which could affect next year's business, becomes important. This section of your marketing plan budget covers important factors that place limits on that plan or forecast opportunities that should be exploited in the coming year: a major new product introduction, new competitor, baby fair or family expos, consolidation with another company or expansion, new distribution outlet, or major change in pricing of classes or services. Although, sometimes it can be difficult to foresee obstacles or opportunities, you can plan for some opportunities as listed above.

Taking a Good Look at the Competition

By using your existing knowledge of other professionals in your community or using websites/Google searches, make a detailed list of your competitors. Once the list is complete, begin to do an overall *competitive analysis* or a "How do you stack up" analysis. This analysis should include complete profiles of your top five competitors. Include in the initial profile the company name, number of partners/employees, location of business, and time in service. Add to the company profiles the prices of services or products. This will give you the range for your own services or products. Evaluate how you want to be viewed in the marketplace: "Low-Price Provider" vs. "High-Price/High-Quality" provider.

Developing Your Tagline

Considering all the information in your business plan, market analysis and competitor profiles, it is time to write your company's *positioning statement* or *tagline*. This positioning statement should be one sentence long that will be used as a tagline on your advertising and promotion. It should be catchy and something that you and your staff can say quickly and concisely. An example would be *"Birthsource.com—Your ONE source for birth and parenting."* This tagline is not only quick and catchy, but also repeats part of the website name within the tagline.

Creating a written marketing plan is only the first step to good business health. Once completed, this plan should be shared with the entire company so that everyone understands the strategies and why resources are being allocated the way they are. Everyone in the company should have some input into the plan and be involved in the measurement or execution of the plan.

But perhaps the most important reason to have a yearly, written marketing plan is that it becomes an important tool for improving your plan year after year. The essence of marketing is to do more of what works and less of what doesn't. Without having clearly established and measurable strategies, you will never learn from your successes and failures.

Networking

Networking has always been a good friend of the new or the small business, but it has become even more user-friendly as a way to reach others. With commitment, your return can be like that of dropping a stone in a lake; the ripple effect can be broad reaching, connecting you to multiple people and clients. It's a great way to establish yourself in your community.

Once you've met, you can use or promote their services and they can do the same for you. Word-of-mouth referrals can mean a lot. Think about it; would you rather trust someone who tells you about a great experience with a business and recommends them, or just the results of an Internet search for businesses who are in close proximity to you? There are many ways that you can network for free or for very little, costing you just time and some extrovertedness.

Chamber of Commerce

Your local Chamber of Commerce can be a gold-mine for a new business. There is often a membership fee, but the benefits will often outweigh the costs. Joining means invitations to well-organized networking events, where you can meet others. In addition to events, some Chambers will offer education-seminars or luncheons on various topics that can help you along as a small business.

U.S. Small Business Association

Visit the sba.gov website and you can click on "Local Assistance". Search for offices that are close to you, resources, and even a calendar of local events for networking. For women entrepreneurs, you can also see what Women Business Centers (WBCs) are closest to you. They specifically cater to women who are just starting and growing their small businesses, providing counseling and training.

Networking Groups

There are many groups you can find online of people that share similar interests with you: fellow small businesses or others looking to networking. Be sure that the group is reputable. You can search for business referral groups in your area. Typically, there is a small monthly fee to join, $10 to $30, but you'll have access to a facilitator of the group as well as a number of local businesses to network and refer, and they'll do the same for you. If you are looking for something less formal, try looking for affinity groups in your area. Some sites, like MeetUp.com, connect you with others in your area with similar interests. Learning from other small businesses and people looking to start their own business can be a great place to learn from those who have advice on what to do, and what to avoid. Learning from others' wisdom can help you to avoid making costly mistakes.

Birth Networks or Community Birth Groups

Perhaps there are already birth professionals meeting in your community. Joining them will bring much information about the birth landscape. If there are no groups of birth professionals meeting

> *Just be a woman's advocate and she will tell all her friends! The other thing I have done is speak to MOPS (Mothers of Preschoolers) groups about my philosophy and services.*
>
> ~*Deb Newton, CNM*

in your community, invite a few that you know to the local coffee shop for an informal meeting. At these meetings, you can share information, and your energy and enthusiasm about what you do.

Marketing You: Writing Your Resume or Curriculum Vitae

If your business card is a small advertisement of who you are, your resume or CV is an infomercial: longer, with more depth and detail. It creates credibility, and entices you to buy, or at least learn more. If you are speaking at a conference or other venue, or looking to submit something for publication, you may be asked to submit a resume or CV.

The main differences between a resume and a CV are the information that is included, the length, and the purpose. A resume is typically one to three pages, and includes education, work history, and skills. It is a concise summary of your experience, typically used when applying for employment. A CV is much longer, with a minimum of two pages, and includes everything a resume contains as well as teaching and research experience, publications, affiliations with organizations, grants/honors/awards, and professional memberships. In Europe, Asia, Middle East, and Africa, most employers will expect a CV. In the United States, a resume is most common, unless you are applying for an academic/scientific/research position, grant, scholarship, or fellowship.

The Resume

Most resumes follow one of two common formats: the work history format or the experiential format. If you have held several jobs that have given you significant experiences and skills, the work history format is probably best. It is essentially a chronological list of your employment from most recent first and then dating back. Each job should include your responsibilities, skills and accomplishments. If you have not held two or more jobs, some elect to use the experiential format, which instead of listing jobs, has skills as the heading with descriptions underneath from any job or position you've held. A word of caution about the experiential format is that it can be confusing to employers, as it is difficult to tell what your work history looks like and what jobs gave you what responsibilities and skills. The work history format, even if you've only held a few jobs, tends to be clearer and easier for another to read and comprehend quickly, which is important! Often, if someone is reading your resume, they will give up quickly and move on to the next person, instead of taking time to decipher it.

Tips for Resumes and CVs

There are many examples of resumes and CVs on the Internet. Search and see what format you like best, both from an aesthetic and organizational standpoint.

Below are some best practices when creating your resume or CV.

1) Be concise.

The information included should be specific, clear, and short. Listed dash items are best. Paragraphs are long-winded and take time to extract the main points.

2) Tailor it.

Periodically, review your resume and make sure it is up to date with all your current information. If you don't keep your resume/CV up to date, you might forget something. Months or years later, it can be hard to remember dates and all the information you want to include. When you need it, it is ready to go, and you can then tailor it to what you need to emphasize. For example, if submitting your resume to speak at a conference on birth, you'll want to ensure that you research the conference, learning objectives, sponsors, and intended audience. Then, on your resume, be sure that you use similar language, and that you highlight your skills and experience to match what the conference is looking for in speakers.

3) Eliminate outdated information and don't repeat information.

If you have stated that you have obtained a certification for a particular profession in the chronological order section of the resume, it does not have to be repeated under education. Be sure that your resume is accurate. There can be serious and even legal ramifications if you are untruthful.

4) *Grammar counts.*

Be sure to use personal pronouns, watch for grammatical errors and changes in verb tense. Do not use the word "I" or "me." Use action verbs to begin the bullet point, or simply list the previous positions, and identify the duties by a higher-level verb. Stay in one tense: usually past or present tense ("served on community service committee").

5) *Be clear.*

Keep in mind that you need to write your resume or CV for someone who likely knows nothing about you or your history. Write out acronyms, explain responsibilities clearly, and use numbers to give context whenever possible. These examples basically say the same thing, but Example 2 gives a broader perspective of work activity.

Example 1

Teaching

I've been teaching couples' classes for 10 years.

Example 2

Childbirth Educator   2004-present

- Certified as an ICEA childbirth educator for 10 years.
- Developed the curriculum for a six-week childbirth education course, refresher course and VBAC class.
- Taught 20 classes for approximately 200 couples as a community / home based educator.
- Acted as an independent educator contracted by Livingston County Memorial Hospital to facilitate 45 classes for approximately 385 couples.

6) *Use action words.*

Using action words helps to show display your skills and to avoid redundancy. See below for some helpful action words that will make your resume pop and seem unique.

7) *Avoid using multiple fonts.*

Stay in one font, such as Times New Roman or Arial Narrow, for the entire resume. Be sure it's a standard font so that anyone with basic software systems will have the same font. Using a non-standard font runs the risk that others won't be able to read it, as it won't open in Word or other programs properly unless sent in a pdf. format.

You'll want you keep your resume consistent and clean. You can use bold italics, and underline to help distinguish sections, but use judiciously. Too many fonts and types can be distracting.

8) Refrain from using clipart or graphics.

It's easy to want to differentiate yourself or spice up your resume, especially if you are very visual or creative. You might look at your one-fonted page of type and think it needs some graphics, but don't be tempted! Graphics can make your resume look unprofessional.

9) Don't undersell yourself!

You'll want to be honest on your resume, but remember that it is a snapshot of all of your work. Be sure to include any work that is relevant and be proud about your accomplishments. Use action words that truly reflect the work that you've done: lead, managed, spearheaded, created. Think of examples of the work you've done and the skills you used in the process, then highlight the skills in your work examples. Use numbers and percentages where you can to show tangible examples.

10) Use fresh eyes.

When you've looked at something long enough, you can become too familiar with it. Remember that a resume must stand on its own, and that a complete stranger will be reading and need to get a clear picture of the skills and experiences. It's a good idea to ask a couple friends or family to review your resume. A fresh set of eyes can catch any small grammatical errors or typos, but can also review to make sure that the content is straightforward and understandable by others.

Writing Your Bio

Current and prospective clients will want to know about the person behind the services or products. When the brick-and-mortar store was replaced by the cold Internet, many missed the personalized touch. Let others know about your professional credentials, as well as any insight into your personal side. Bios are helpful on websites and social media platforms. The length and how much you share depends on what the bio is for, and how comfortable you are with sharing.

It's a good idea to write several versions: a very short, medium, and longer bio, so that you have multiple forms of it on hand, depending on the purpose. Remember that the bio should be comprised mostly of professional information with a dash of personal at the end. Start with your name and write in third person.

Here are some things you could consider including:

1. Number of years in the field

2. Where you are originally from and where you live now

3. Your current position and relevant past positions/experiences

4. Your goal or philosophy around your work/passions

5. Personality at the end: hobbies, family, etc...

6. A picture, typically a headshot. It could a professional or an informal headshot depending on who the audience is.

WorkSheet III

Marketing Budget

List all possible items needed for marketing your business and approximate cost.

Item	Quantity	Cost per Item
Total Cost:		

Who is your target market?

_____

_____

_____

_____

_____

_____

_____

_____

_____

_____

How will you reach your target market?

_____

_____

_____

_____

_____

_____

_____

_____

Have you changed the name of your business from Chapter 1? If so, write it here and sketch a logo to accompany the company name.

_____

Write a positioning statement or tagline for your business.

_____
_____
_____
_____
_____

Write four marketing objectives.

_____
_____
_____
_____
_____
_____
_____
_____
_____
_____
_____

List the top three marketing tools you plan to use.

_____

_____

_____

_____

_____

_ _

_ _

Who are your five competitors? What are their strengths and weaknesses?

_____

_____

_____

_____

_____

_____

_____

_____

_____

_____

_____

_____

_____

_____

How many hospitals or birth centers are in your community? List their names, addresses and main phone numbers.

_____

_____

_____

_____

_____

_____

_____

_____

_____

_____

How many babies are born each year in your community?

_____

How many other birth professionals are offering the same services as you?

_____

_____

_____

_____

How will/does your company differ from others in the community (include features and benefits)?

_____

_____

_____

_____

_____

_____

_____

- -

_____

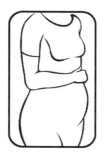

Chapter 4

Advertising

If you do build a great experience, customers tell each other about that. Word of mouth is very powerful.

—Jeff Bezos

There is an old adage; "you have to spend money to make money." While many in the birth community consider their work as a passion, it is important to understand that it is only fair to be paid for a day's work. Who pays you? Your customers or clients. How will your customers know you are there without advertising? Media is the method used to convey advertising messages. There are three main types of advertising media: broadcast (radio and TV), electronic (email, websites, e-newsletters), and print (brochures, flyers, newspaper advertisements, etc). In this chapter, we are going to focus on the two easiest and most inexpensive: electronic and print media.

Developing Your Logo

Drive along any road in the U.S. or Canada, and you will see recognizable logos: the golden arches of McDonalds, the green goddess of Starbucks, the sunrise of Days Inn, the red cowboy hat of Arby's, or the red logo of Dairy Queen. A logo brings instant recognition to any goods or services that are provided. In the birth business, logo recognition can be seen with ICEA, DONA International, and Lamaze International. These logos are generally well-recognized and are used on all communications generated by these organizations.

When selecting a logo, remember the focus of your business. Logos for birth doulas might include an image of a pregnant belly, hands, or babies. More abstract logos, such as a labyrinth (depicting a journey or mother/child), may also be used and can represent a diverse group of practitioners who are working together. Native American/American Indian symbols, without any modifications, may be used if permission of the tribe is obtained. Trees of life, with wording "hidden" in the tree leaves and the trunks of the trees depicting a woman's body outline, have also been used with success.

Teddy bears and rattles are attractive for new parents, and depict light and playful messages. Postpartum specialists, such as doulas or lactation educators/ consultants, may choose images of families, and lactation experts prefer abstract images of a mother nursing her baby.

Logos are not only a depiction of your company, but they become a memory hook. People will remember them, no matter how they are displayed: on a website, blog, business card, brochure, and car decal. Instant recognition is something to strive for when designing and adopting a logo for your business.

Electronic Media

Once you are happy with a recognizable logo, it is time to begin putting that logo on a series of advertising media. E-newletters and blogs are a fun and easy way to reach large numbers of people with thoughts and ideas

An e-newsletter can be created by a company (such as Constant Contact, www.constantcontact.com) that will keep track of your email database. For one low fee per month, you will be able to generate professional looking newsletters with the ease of using Microsoft Word. For a few dollars more, the ability to upload numerous photos, or access their stock photo library, allows you to make your newsletter more visually appealing and eye-catching. Some opt for writing their email newsletters as a true email and sending the email to a "gang" of email addresses in the "bcc," or *blind copy*, area of the address block of the email. Generally, it is unadvisable to do this, as web companies will be tracking gang emails and may soon identify your email address/website as one that sends out spam. It may be best to go with an e-newsletter company.

Websites

A website is a collection of written information, images, videos or other digital information hosted on one or several web servers. Literally anyone can create a website today. Anyone. When teaching clients or consumers about evidence-based information on the web, suggest that they go beyond looking at the person's credentials and investigate the true origins of the author's information. If the information is footnoted and quoted from reputable references, then chances are, the information is credible.

Websites today can be critical to the success or failure to your business. A website serves many purposes; it is the modern-day equivalent to the yellow pages or newspaper advertisement. It also allows your other advertising material to be less cluttered and more eye catching, promising your target market more, if they go to your website. It is your calling card. It is how people get to know you and your product. For some, it is the test on whether a business is really legitimate.

Consider which company you would feel more comfortable to give your money: Company A, which has advertisements with a phone number, or Company B, which has advertisements with a website where you can learn more about the owners, history of the business, read reviews of current customers, and see that they are supported by the Better Business Bureau? Unlike purchasing a normal day-to-day item, like a watch or toothpaste, purchasing a service or product connected with a child will cause parents to do a lot of research. Before trusting a company with the well-being of their child, they'll want to know as much as they can about you!

A webpage is a document, often written in HTML (HyperTex Markup Language), which describes the structure of text-based information in a document--by denoting certain text as headings, bold, italics, paragraphs, lists, and so on—and to supplement that text with *interactive forms, embedded images*, and other objects.

A web browser is a software application that enables a user to display and interact with text, images, and other information typically located on a webpage at a website on the Internet. Examples of browsers include Google Chrome, Firefox, and Internet Explorer. The pages of a website can be accessed through a common root URL (Uniform Research Locator) or "address." A URL would look like this: www.vbac.com.

Visit other websites and take note of features that you like and don't like. What makes you want to return? Those features are the ones you will want to make note.

Consider having someone create your website. While there are many free websites locations, and also web design programs, look at a minimum of three designers. Also, assess your budget and know how much you can spend on web design. When you walk in to talk to a web designer, you can have ideas. Print off some designs, color combinations, and more to show the designer what you prefer. Visit the designers' site, look at his / her portfolio and talk to their clients for advice on how service is provided. Is there 24/7 tech support? How do you reach them? Does the cost include only design? Hosting? Is there an incremental cost for small changes or adjustments? What would be your monthly fee?

Christopher James is the owner of Websource LLC and is an experienced web designer. He has created a list of five things you might consider when making the important decision to have a website. Chris says web design companies should SERVE you:

1) Skill

Different designers have different skills. For example, if you want to build a website with ecommerce capability, this requires a completely different skill set than a strictly informational website. Ask for examples of websites they have built that are similar in features to your requirements.

2) Experience

Ask how long they have been in business. Many website design companies come and go, but the answer to this question might be a good indicator as to whether they are going to be available when you need future updates. Most companies will also publish a portfolio of work. Take the time to look through it.

3) Relationship

How pleasant are they to communicate with? Do they return your emails/calls promptly? Do they take the time to explain things to you in layman's terms? Remember, you are likely looking at a long-term relationship with the company you choose.

4) Value

The cost of a website will depend largely on the complexity of the work involved, but pricing can also vary tremendously from one company to another. Shop around! Expect to pay a deposit of 30% to 50%.

5) Examples

"Build it and they will come" does NOT apply to the web, at least not without SEO (Search Engine Optimization) and other e-marketing strategies. Not every website designer is a marketing specialist, and websites that fail to attract traffic are unlikely to succeed. Ask for specific examples of how they have helped past customers.

See more tips from Christopher James at the end of this chapter.

Print Media

Print ads are effective in reaching a select market. A birth-business owner may place print ads in small community newspapers, natural health magazines, or health-related newsletters or papers. Print ads can also be placed in focused magazines, journals, or conference manuals. These focused ads tend to be expensive and have limited exposure to your target market.

Sizes of print ads vary from 2" x 3.5" or business card size to ¼ page, ½ page, or full page. The choice may also be horizontal or vertical, in black/white or color.

Table Tents

Table tents are similar to a brochure, except they have a slightly different format and are made to sit upright on tables. Many software packages have a template for making table tents. Be concise with a graphic or catchphrase that will attract a client to read more, and use a thicker card stock paper that will be durable and look nice, even after multiple people have handled your tent.

Use your local resources. Often, you can work with local businesses to make advertising deals that are very reasonable. Perhaps a local coffee shop will allow you to have table tents on their tables for a month while you have a stack of their advertisements sitting out at your business. Larger companies will often need to sift through bureaucracy and forms and approvals in order to consider deals. Local small businesses have a bond; they are often closer to members of the community and work hard to obtain business. A good resource is to go on your city's website and search out local or small businesses. Make a list of the ones that you think would be a positive business to have clients connect with your business. For example, if you are an aromatherapist, soliciting a candle shop to advertise in may be the perfect combination.

Business Cards

Even with all of the Internet marketing available, it is sometimes effective to use business cards. There has been quite a transition in business card printing in the last 10 years. Previously, only office supply stores or stationers could supply business cards. Then, with the advent of more economical computer printers, self-printed business cards with micro-perfed edged appeared. Now with companies such as www.vistaprint.com , www.gotprint.net, www.123print.com, www.zazzle.com , www.moo.com, and others, professionally printed and double-sided business cards are not only economical, but fun to create online. Many of these companies also offer online design of brochures.

> *I never pass up an opportunity to tell people about what I do. I always have either my business cards or a pen and paper with me. Don't ever be afraid to start up a conversation. I've met new clients at my gym, at work, at school, in the grocery store, etc. Enthusiasm is catching so I spread it around. I've gotten several clients because a family member or friend has mentioned me to someone they know.*
>
> *~Jamilla Walker, RN*
> *Doula, childbirth educator,*
> *and midwife-to-be*

Business cards can be used in a variety of ways. The obvious is giving out to clients or when you meet someone, giving them your business card as they may be a potential client or know a client they want to recommend to you. Consider also using the back of the business card. With a little extra work or a few dollars, you can have some basic bullet points on the back of your business card. It instantly becomes a mini advertising tool. Also, chat with local businesses, as they sometimes have areas or posting boards where you can leave or tack up your business cards.

Handouts and Brochures

Handouts are one of the most important items of a birth-related business; they last longer than the personal interaction and meet the needs of the visual learner. To help you create the very best handouts, this section is divided into four basic areas: content, illustrations, design, and reproduction.

By *Content*, we mean the text: the words that are printed on the paper. Begin with basic ideas and progress to an outline. Take the time to outline your brochure. See if it makes sense as a whole before you begin putting too much effort into individual paragraphs. Always, always allow someone else to proofread for clarity and errors. Consider writing using a question-and- answer format. It's often easy to recall the typical questions, and a very effective handout can be made once you've written the questions out, answered them, then sorted the information into a logical order.

Limit the objective/topic of each handout. A key step to writing a good brochure is remembering your audience. Many handouts and articles are written on a 5th-grade level for best understanding. If your handout is going to focus on cesarean birth, don't include information about vaginal births after cesarean or VBACs. That is another handout topic.

On any piece of print material, remember TEAM: The Essential Advertising Messages. Often, this will depend on how big your print material is and the goal. If you are making a postcard to mail out or give away, you can only include so much information without it looking cluttered. Your goal is to entice your target market to want to learn more, perhaps by visiting your website or your place of business. If you are creating a brochure, you can include more material. Your goal is to inform and give background. Your TEAM begins with the basics: name of your business, what you do, and how people can obtain your products or services. The rest of the content or the graphics should complement and enhance your advertisement, not muddle it.

Illustrations are pictures or drawings that make the information easier to understand and remember. Too much text may be boring or intimidating. Too many illustrations may distract from the impact of the handout. Illustrations should break up text and add color, allowing the reader's eye to rest and set the tone of the handout. Again, if you are creating a cesarean birth handout, an illustration where the expectant mother appears somewhat frightened, and there appears to be blood in the IV fluid, is not the one to use. While expectant mothers may have fear about cesareans, and may even have transfusions, this is not the first impression you'll want to give to the students in your class. When editing illustrations with Microsoft Paint or another program, be sure to crop out any white space, especially if your background is a color other than white.

Need photographs to include in brochures and handouts but you are not a great photographer? A great place to get photos is www.istockphoto.com. With a small membership fee and a small fee per photo, you can add excitement and interest to your business brochure, informational handouts, and more. Want to create something with humor? An exciting website to create interesting graphics is www.imagechef.com. Free with limited capability, this website allows you to take ordinary items, such as pizza boxes or freeway signs, and put your own information on those signs. Remember that what you create impacts your business as you create memorable, and sometimes humorous signs and graphics.

Design is the glue that brings together the text and the illustrations. Some handouts and brochures are read. Others are opened, quickly scanned, and then filed away. The first impression is very important.

Color can be used in illustrations, design elements (lines, bars, etc.), the paper, and/or the ink. Using color can have an enormous impact, but remember; sometimes using just a bit of it is more effective than color everywhere.

Your text is made more readable when short words, short sentences, short paragraphs, and white space are creatively used.

Desktop computers have made it easier than ever to quickly switch back and forth between different type styles (known as fonts). Be careful. Just as with the use of color, less is usually more. Be careful using the fancy fonts that are available. For a party announcement, they're fine. For an education handout, they are inappropriate. Keep with simple fonts, such as Times New Roman, Arial, Verdana, or Century Gothic.

By *Production*, we mean making copies affordably. There are several alternatives for the cost-wise creator: print it yourself on a home computer printer, have color copies printed at a printing company, or purchase pre-illustrated paper from an office store or online company, such as Paper Direct (www.paperdirect.com), or design completely online at www.vistaprint.com. Prior to printing, Vistaprint will send a pdf. proof copy for your approval.

Work with standard-sized sheets of paper. Start visualizing your handout or brochure by folding or stapling familiar paper sizes. Take a sheet of regular 8.5" by 11" paper and fold it in half or thirds, and see if your vision will fit this format. Begin writing your text on this sample brochure or handout. Make certain you have enough space to say exactly what you need or want to say.

Pre-illustrated papers are great because the expensive color printing is already done. Purchasers can buy a package of sheets, and use only the black ink of a printer to add their message. The result is a full-color handout.

10 Ways to Promote Your Website

Christopher James, Websource, LLC

1. Your website should be mobile-friendly, and responsive.

We all know the use of mobile devices has been skyrocketing over the past few years. If you're not familiar with "Responsive Design," look it up. Responsive websites not only give you a great viewing experience, regardless of device or screen resolution, but Google loves them.

2. Stop worrying about SEO, and start writing quality content.

Once upon a time, if you wanted to increase your rankings, you simply crammed your website full of keywords. Smart website owners know that while this might have attracted visitors, it was never an effective strategy for converting visitors into sales. Write quality content, however, and those readers will turn into repeat visitors, and into sales.

3. Stop worrying about Search Engines, and start worrying about SEO.

To clarify, a lot of garbage has been written about search engine optimization. Search engines are much better at grading websites than they used to be, and chances are, if your website has good content, you're doing okay. However, if you want to maximize your website's potential, you do still need your website to be "optimized." Find a local website developer and talk to them about making sure you have a well-coded website, and that the basics of SEO are done right.

4. Use Social Media.

Social media is a great way engage with your customers and colleagues. But it's not for everyone, and not all businesses will benefit equally. While building Facebook pages or Twitter accounts are "free," they still require a lot of time and effort to be worthwhile. Study your competition, and see what works and does not work for them. Remember, social media is not about you, and it's not about selling your product or service. It's about engaging in conversation and building relationships.

5. Think local.

Searching for local businesses online is up, but did you know that Google, Yahoo, and Bing all have separate local directories that are free to sign up for? Other local directories, such as Yellow Pages, also have free basic listings. Local websites, like DaytonLocal.com, can help drive traffic to your website. Look for these local websites where you are.

6. Start a company blog.

Writing articles about your business or your industry can be a great way to drive traffic to your website, and increase your search engine visibility to boot. Be sure to commit to a blog before you start. Blogs are often started with great enthusiasm, but then neglected shortly afterwards. A blog that hasn't been updated in months often looks worse than not having a blog at all.

7. Increase back-links.

Ask other website owners to consider linking to your website. Google, in particular, views the number of incoming links to your website in your favor. One-way links are more valuable, but reciprocal linking is good, provided the website in question is a quality site.

8. Start a mailing list. But never send unsolicited emails.

A legitimate mailing list made up of your customers can be invaluable. But no matter how good your intentions, or how well you present your emails, you risk becoming blacklisted if you send unsolicited emails. Never buy mailing lists. If you want to start a legitimate mailing list, use a legitimate service, like Constant Contact or Mail Chimp, who will ensure you comply with the law.

9. Solicit the advice of your web developer. But never respond to unsolicited emails.

Do you ever get emails offering you help with SEO and marketing your website? Any email from an unsolicited source that wants to add your website to thousands of search engines, or to help in any way with marketing your business is bad news. If they use SPAM to promote their services, can you really trust them? Talk to your website developer about legitimate ways to help promote your website.

10. Use your website!

This may seem obvious, but if you have a website, your URL (website address) should appear anywhere you instinctively put your telephone number, from business cards to brochures to offline advertising to vehicle decals.

Christopher James is the owner of Web-source LLC, and has been building successful websites for local businesses in Ohio since 2001. Chris is married to Molly and the proud father of two boys. You can visit Chris on the web at www.websourcellc.com.

WorkSheet 4

Marketing/Ad Assessment

Your first two marketing strategies: where you will obtain them, and where you plan to distribute them.

_____

_____

_____

_____

_____

_____

_____

_____

Your second two marketing strategies: where you will obtain them, and where you plan to distribute them.

_____

_____

_____

_____

_____

_____

_____

How Your Competitors Market and Advertise

Name	How Long in Business	Services Offered	Strengthz	Weakness	Marketing

How Your Competitors Market and Advertise

Method of Advertising	Usage (where distributed)	Rated (potential income)
Business Cards		
Brochure		
Postcards		
Flyers		
Brochures		
Ads		
Health fairs		
Writing Articles		
Public Speaking		
Press Releases		
Website		
Blog		
Facebook		
Memes/Infographics		
Direct Referrals		
Networking		
Word of Mouth		

Name and location of hospitals, physician offices, and other locations to distribute business cards, flyers, or brochures.

Name	Address, City, State, Zip

Sample Press Release

Contact information
Name
Address
City, State, Zip
Phone/Fax/Email

(Release Date)
For Immediate Release

Catchy Headline

City where this happens. This is the body of the press release. Usually a press release has three paragraphs, on one page. Wording is usually conversational. At the bottom of the page, end the press release with the word "END," "30," or "###." This signals the end of the press release. The first paragraph tells the reader what the writer wants them to know.

The second paragraph is extra information, and may include quotations from speakers or interesting tidbit information

The third paragraph is summing up what you have already told the reader with an emphasis on how to reach someone for additional information, including phone numbers and email addresses.

END

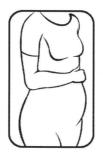

Chapter 5

140 is the New 411

Social Networking is the word of mouth of the 21st Century.

—Heather Livingston

One of the most inexpensive ways of marketing today is social media marketing. Social media marketing, also known as social influence marketing, is using social media platforms and communities (such as blogs, Twitter, and Facebook) to promote and advertise. In essence, the advertiser no longer has a one way conversation with a potential customer; they can have a two-way conversation. In using social media marketing, it is important to understand the Four C's: content, context, connections and conversation.

Content is the actual information that is being given to the consumer: blog posts, video, podcasts, photos, status updates on Facebook, or information with a web link via Twitter. *Context* is the tool used: website, blog, etc. Sharing content enables the *connec-*

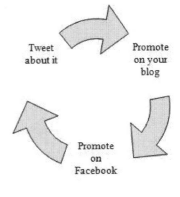

Tweet about it

Promote on your blog

Promote on Facebook

tions: finding people with similar interests or professions, such as maternity nurses, midwives, lactation consultants, doulas or childbirth educators. Finally, *conversations* between the originator of the information and those with whom they've connected.

These can take the form of blog comments, Twitter replies, or even Retweets (repeating what someone posts on Twitter), or writing on a person's wall on Facebook. It is through these conversations that the person-to-person link is made.

Social media marketing has become the new word-of-mouth marketing. Brian Tracy said fully 84% of sales in America take place as a result of word-of-mouth advertising. Some of the most important sales activities are those that take place between customers and prospects, between friends and colleagues in the forms of advice, and recommendations on what to buy or not buy and who to buy from.

Why should you consider using social media marketing to promote your business? One reason is demographics: 74% of social media users are women between the ages of 28 and 59. Here are four more reasons why you should consider using social media:

1. It's current. Your website/blog is exposed to large groups of people in a spontaneous fashion.

This is the newest way of communication, and many people are visiting these social websites and communities.

2. It's personal.

The visitor can put a name and some selected personal information to a business. This makes their contact with you much more intimate than an ad. It becomes the voice of the company. In turn, the company can listen to those who respond to promotions.

3. Its low-cost/high returns.

If done by yourself, costs are limited to only time. The benefits will often exceed the cost. It would take you thousands of dollars to buy many links; social media has the ability to give you that for free and it's flexible. You can make changes quickly and easily. Basically, you reduce overall marketing expenses.

4. It complements other efforts.

Social media optimization and marketing is usually community-specific. It doesn't interfere with any other methods of getting traffic to your website. It can and will fit perfectly with an advertising campaign targeting other websites or search engines. Nearly 81% of users state that social media efforts generated exposure for their business by improving traffic to websites and building new partnerships.

> *I use a blog platform for a combined website and blog. Many of the pages have static content with information about my classes, fees, etc, but I update the blog section about once a week. I've found that the continually new content keeps my previous clients coming back to my site on a regular basis and thus keeps my birth business fresh in their minds for referring their friends. In addition, over 50% of my clients hire me solely from finding me via my website. I highly recommend having a good one.*
>
> *~Molly Remer*
> *Talk Birth, Rolla, Missouri, talkbirth. wordpress.com*

There are four basic types of social media (we will talk about a few of these):

Social Bookmarking: Pinterest, Del.icio.us

Social News: Digg, Reddit

Social Networking: Facebook, Twitter, Linkedin

Social Photo and Video Share: YouTube, Flickr, Instagram (exclusively mobile)

Psychologists, parents and some professionals are concerned that spending so much time on social media is an example of media addiction. While this may be true, individuals who spend a large portion of their day online do reap some rewards. According to social media researcher Paul Zak, *oxytocin* release percentages are in *double digits* when using Facebook and Twitter. It is, therefore, gratifying to have your Facebook status "liked" or "shared," or to have your Tweet retweeted.

What are blogs and why do you would want one with an RSS feed?

A blog is a publication of content and web links, sorted in chronological order, with the most recent entry at the top. The content of the blog entries reflects personal or company interests. The word blog is a *portmanteau*, or the fusion, of two words (web and log) together to make a new word. One might call it a diary in reverse. While the concept of the "noun" blog is only 11 years old, "blog" can also be used as a verb, meaning to *maintain or add content to a blog*, or it can be a noun, blogger, as someone who maintains a blog. Much like a website, a blog can include not only text, but images and links to other blogs or websites. A blog can also include music, videos, and podcasting. Blogs came a part of the mainstream media in 2001, when blogging became a political catharsis.

Blogenomics are affordable, yet blogs are editorially unchecked. While blogs can be set up for free by anyone, there is an element of lack of editorial supervision. This means that good writers, mediocre writers, and even bad writers can blog. No one has control over content, grammar, or evidence-based research vs. opinion.

Blog entries can be a passion you are excited about on one day, or they can be a photo (as long as you have explicit permission to post it), or even a video (for example, from YouTube). Perhaps a better definition of a blog is a diary entry that everyone has access to, and the purpose of your diary is to promote your business.

Two popular ways to create blogs are wordpress. org and www.blogspot.com. For Wordpress, you need to download the program and find a host for the blog. At Google's Blogspot, all of the software is on the Internet, and you can either write directly online and then publish, or write your blog entry in a word processing document, such as Word and then cut and paste into Blogspot. Both of these formats allow for you to post photos, blog entries, videos, plus have an assortment of "gadgets" along the side of the blog entry itself. These gadgets may include a photo of the blogger, their favorite websites or blogs, and company updates (especially helpful if they are trainers or workshop presenters).

On Blogspot, you can track the traffic by day, month, and all time. This can come as a written report or graphic. Traffic stats can tell the country, referring URL (such as Google), and even what equipment the visitor is using (PC or Apple).

Updating a blog can be daily, several times a week, weekly, or even several times per month. A blogger will have more followers if he/she blogs more frequently, and blogs about cutting-edge issues. In our business, blogging about current events, such as new research or events, such as World Breastfeeding Week (in August), are highly sought after.

RSS is Rich Site Summary or Really Simple Syndication, and is a format for delivering regularly changing web content. It is an easy way to distribute headlines, update notices, and some content to a large number of people. For example, if a blog has an RSS feed, those who frequently check the blog can be updated when the blog is updated, rather than tediously check back to see if the blog has been updated.

Facebook Is for Kids, Tweens, and Teens, right?

Not exactly! A growing number of baby boomers and younger are accessing this social media. Beginning on February 4, 2004 Mark Zuckerberg launched Facebook as an exclusive social network for Harvard students. Within four months, Facebook had added 30 more college networks. Today, it is estimated that Facebook is the 2nd most valuable Internet company. According to Zuckerberg, Facebook now has 1.9 billion active users with more than 728 million users logging on to Facebook at least once each day: a 48% increase from 2010 to 2011. More than two-thirds of Facebookers are outside of college, with the 35+ year olds being the fastest growing demographic.

In the age range for childbearing, an estimated 87.9 million individuals are on Facebook, with the highest traffic time being mid-week between 1 p.m. and 3 p.m. in each time zone. Thus, if you desire an international reach to your business, you should be prepared to update Facebook very frequently.

Facebook allows for both B2B (business-to-business) and B2C (business-to-customer) interaction. By using the four C's of social media, an entrepreneur can successfully link a website, Facebook page, Twitter account, and blog together so potential customers will see a full range of products, services, and philosophies.

No longer is a business a one-dimensional entity. It has a personality, likes/dislikes, and a Facebook page!

Users of Facebook can choose fan pages according to their interests to connect and interact with others with like-minded interests. Thus, birth practitioners can join fan pages of *The Business of Being Born, Orgasmic Birth*, and other birth-related, and non-birth-related businesses.

Facebook is free to users, but generates revenue from advertising, including banner ads (a banner ad is an ad embedded into a web page and linking to another webpage). Each user has a *wall*, or timeline, that allows friends to post messages for the user to see, very much like graffiti. Friends can poke another friend, letting them know they thought about them. The *status* part of the page allows users to inform friends and visitors about their activities of the day or week.

Photos can be uploaded and separated into albums, increasing the social sharing quality of Facebook. Facebook Notes was introduced in 2006 for the importation and promotion of blogs. Two years later, a type of instant messaging, called "Chat," was introduced, allowing users to have short bursts of conversations similar to text or instant messaging. "Chat" has now become Messenger.

How can you blend high-touch aspects with Facebook? Personalizing the timeline cover can be both high touch and a great marketing tool. Visiting timeline cover websites, such as www.timelinecoverbanner.com, enables even the novice the opportunity to create an interesting and eye-catching timeline cover.

Expressing your feelings through emoticons, endearing photos, and memes can allow your "friends" to get to know you, and you will feel more personal to them. Additionally, wishing your Facebook friends happy birthday, or congratulating them on an accomplishment, also adds a high-touch component.

Twitter, Tweeting, and Tweets

Twitter is another social media, but one that is a real-time short messaging service. Started in San Francisco in 2006, Twitter's popularity grew exponentially. By asking the simple question, "What are you doing?" and allowing only 140 characters to answer, Twitter allows followers to see what is happening to those whom they follow via mobile texting, instant message, or the web.

TweetDeck is a personal browser for staying in touch with what is happening now and interfaces with Twitter and Facebook. A free download, TweetDeck allows the user to update both Twitter and Facebook simultaneously, but still with the 140 characters. With TweetDeck, retweeting (repeating a message or quote from someone so that people who follow you will see it too) is as easy as the click of a mouse. With Tweet-Deck, you can see friends' Facebook status changes, and add several other columns that are specific to your interests.

To link your Facebook status updates to your Twitter account, on the website of the application you want to connect (Facebook), find the button/link asking you to connect your Twitter account (usually "Connect to Twitter"). On Facebook, this is located in the General Settings section, then under App Settings. You'll be directed to a Twitter website asking you to log in to your Twitter account. Check that it's secure by verifying the URL starts with https://twitter.com. After logging in, Twitter will ask you to approve the application. Be sure to review the various permissions you are granting to the application. These are listed in green (what the app can do with your account), and red (what the app can't do). Click "Authorize app" if you'd like to connect. Your Facebook status will now be placed as a Tweet simultaneously.

Twitter and TweetDeck both use TinyURL™ and bit.ly. TinyURL™ makes long URLs useable, and they don't break when sending to the recipient. What may at one time have been a URL of 25 to 30 characters is condensed to a URL that would look something like this: http://tinyurl.com/childbirth. Bit.ly also allows users to shorten, share, and track URLs.

LinkedIn: The Professionals' Facebook

LinkedIn, like other social media, came into being in the early 2000s. Now a publicly traded company, it boasts 225 million members in over 10 offices worldwide. Touted as the "professionals' Facebook," LinkedIn is much more than photos of your cat, or what you made for dinner. LinkedIn allows the member to promote their professional history as well as their current activity. Employers do check LinkedIn before hiring new prospects.

Through LinkedIn, your contacts can "endorse" you for skills, adding to your professional image. This can be particularly helpful when, and if, you are job searching. In the birth-related field, skills can include "birth," "babies," "health care" "holistic care," and "childbirth." The more contacts and endorsements you have, the more appealing you become.

Members of LinkedIn have the option to upgrade from the free account to paid accounts that have additional features. Work with the free account for a while and then see if the upgrades are worth the money.

So, why would a birth professional want to use blogs, Facebook, Twitter, or LinkedIn? It all goes back to the basis of marketing. It takes a certain number of exposures from potential customers to make them actual customers. By using blogs, Facebook, and Twitter to keep your business, services, and products in front of your potential customers' focus, you will increase the chances of making them your actual customers in much less time. This is marketing in the 21st century.

Pinterest

Have you ever made a scrapbook or browsed through one? Pinterest is the new generation of scrapbooking. Create your own online board and pin things that you like. You can search for things on Pinterest in multiple categories, or you can pin from the Internet. Link to your friends to see the pins they post or let them see yours. It's a great way to easily find out about new products or websites, and it's another way you can promote your business and your technological savvy. Informative pins, with how-to's or tips, are 30% more engaging than other pins. Promote your products or services and see what people pin in order to assess what is trending and popular.

The Pinterest website is easy to navigate for business use, and provides a step-by-step from how to make items on your site "pinable," to learning how you can use tools such as Pinterest Analytics to explore the metrics of how many people post, what they are posting from you, and the demographics of the pinners so you know what clients and customers have interest in, and what you can focus on to deliver them more of the content and products they want. Pinterest is very visual. The pictures catch the viewer's eyes first, so you'll want to ensure that your images are crisp, clear, alluring and professional. For some, text is best, for others, seeing the visuals is much more captivating and attractive.

Instagram

A picture is worth a thousand words, and Instagram is the perfect example of how today's generation want images and photos to do the talking. Instagram is the photographer's Facebook. Instagramers can follow businesses or individuals, or search for pictures to view or repost onto their own profile. Video clips and images become the center focus, and if you follow a business, sometimes you feel like a VIP, knowing about new products, services, or sales before anyone else.

With an image or video, a little text, and some hashtags, you can link to the over 300 million active daily users of Instagram. Looking to be international with your business? Because Instagram isn't just for Americans. Over 70% of users live in countries outside of the United States, so it's likely that your followers won't just be in your country, but you'll have a global reach to a diverse audience.

You might be thinking, how powerful can images be for my business? There are many success stories that prove just that. When Ben & Jerry's launched a new flavor, 17% more people became aware from Instagram. Remember that if you combine multiple platforms on social media, you can exponentially increase the positive results. Mercedes Benz used Facebook and Instagram together. The result from this dynamic duo? A 54% increase in visits to their website. The pen might be mightier than the sword, but the photograph might have just become the mightiest.

Time Commitment to Social Media Marketing

According to Michael A. Stelzner, there is a direct relationship between how long marketers have been using social media and their weekly time commitment. People just beginning usually commit about two hours per week, learning their way around the individual site, and what all can be done interactively with other social media being used (such as how to post blog entries on a Facebook page).

After a few months, however, the average jumped to 10 hours per week. It is believed that with time, more blog followers, more Twitter followers, and more friends on Facebook take more time to read and update. They then share what they have found with connections and friends: retweeting and reposting. Therefore, it is vital to schedule enough time to be effective, yet not so much time that nothing else gets done.

Privacy, Etiquette, and Social Networking

Everyone sees what you post on the Internet. Everyone. When representing your company and your passion, you must remember that everyone can see, copy, and refer to your post. Generally speaking, too, be cautious about putting too much information, especially *personal* information, such as phone numbers, addresses, or specific family or business information, etc.

Explore the relationship between social media and HIPAA, the Health Insurance Portability and Accountability Act. This law protects the confidentiality and security of health care information. Be mindful of professional boundaries, which become less clear online. It is best to treat social media like a crowd in an elevator; if you wouldn't say something in a crowded elevator, you should not say it on social media. One birth organization, the International Childbirth Education Association, has developed a position paper about social media and HIPAA. You can find the link to this position paper in the reference section of this book.

When using social media marketing to promote your business, give information or make statements that promote your business, not detract from it. For example, a birth professional who constantly updates their Facebook status with depressing comments about life or complaints, will not be building quality connections. Consider whose photo is posted on Facebook, your blog, or a website, and make certain a *Permission to Photograph* is on file (a sample photo release form is at the end of Chapter 2).

You do not have to Tweet every hour, blog every day, or update a Facebook status at every turn. It is okay to not say anything. Actually, silence makes people interested in what has been happening since the last entry!

A Word about Memes and Infographics

A *meme* (pronounced *meem*), first described by Richard Dawkins in his 1976 book, *The Selfish Gene,* is an idea, behavior, or style that spreads from person to person within a culture. An Internet meme is an image with an interesting comment that mimics reality, such as a photo of Grumpy Cat with the words, "Unnecessary medical interventions? I don't think so," written on the photo. Memes can be created through programs, such as PowerPoint, that allows the creator to apply text over photos, or through websites, such as www.memegenerator.net. A meme can be a humorous tool to make a point, and can easily be shared around Facebook and other social media.

Just like other Social Media, memes should follow etiquette, and not be attacking or unpleasant. The meme can be creative, ironic, or funny. Additionally, be aware of copyright infringements for photos, illustrations, or graphics used in memes.

Information graphics, or infographics, are the newest way to disseminate information on social media in a concise and visually appealing way to attract a larger audience. While infographics have been around for many years (well, since 1626), the increased usage by Facebook, Twitter, Pinterest, and Instagram have brought infographics to a whole new level. Birth-related organizations, such as MANA, Amnesty International, ICEA, ICAN, AHWONN, and Lamaze International, have all used infographics to promote new studies, interesting data, or new campaigns. Three of the popular and free sites at which to make infographics are www.venngage.com, www.infographicreator.com, and www.piktochart.com.

What Are QR Codes?

QR Codes (or Quick Response Codes) might well be the grandfather of the UPC code that is now on most items we purchase. Developed in 1960 by the Japanese who wished to make grocery inventory and check-out easier, today these square barcodes can be captured by a smartphone camera and app. It can contain up to 7,000 characters, and are used to track products or take a consumer to a specific website. In marketing, however, QR codes allow the consumer to access a website without entering in the URL into the browser; just scan the picture.

Created on QR Code generator websites (such as, www.qrstuff.com) and saved as a jpg., these boxy graphics can be used on business cards, postcards, brochures, or even on other websites if you need to link to your other online offerings. Literally, it takes less than five minutes to create a QR Code. Nearly as fast as you type in the URL or web address, the generator will create your QR Code. Then you can download it to your computer, print it, or email it.

To read the QR Code with a smart phone or tablet, the QR Code Reader App from places, such as iTunes or Google Play, must be loaded onto the device. Once the QR Code is centered in the middle of a camera-type display from the Reader App, recognition takes place and the app takes you to the URL associated with the Code.

A Final Word: What are Skype and Google Hangout?

Networking is a vital piece to keeping the birth community energized. With the world-wide appeal of Facebook and Twitter, occasionally it is important to reach out personally and interact with other professionals, either in a casual setting or webinar or other professional setting. Skype and Google Hangout are the best options for this type of in-person interaction.

Knowing what you want from a platform, such as Skype or Google Hangout, will help you determine which one to download. If you want to make calls or text, then use Skype. If you want to talk to large groups, Google Hangout is free, but Skype has a fee. Both allow you to share your computer screen, but only with Google Hangout can you prepare and test before inviting people to share a look.

Skype

Skype can be a noun, when referring to the telecommunications software program that allows for either spoken or video enhanced conversations over the Internet. Skype can be a verb when explaining the act of using the Internet for these conversations. Part of the Microsoft family, Skype can include text messaging, voice, and video calls using Internet access, the free program or app, and a device with a camera and microphone (computer, smartphone, or smart tablet). There are many free services within the Skype program, as well as expanded services, for which you will pay a fee. For example, you can Skype with up to 10 people (as long as one is a Skype Premium member) for generally $4.99 for 12 months and $7.49 for 3 months.

Founded in 2003 in Denmark, Skype has millions of users worldwide. This is mostly due to the ease with which Skype can be used. Most of the Skype commands are simple point-and-click in answer to the various prompts. From video calls, to group video calls, to file sharing, Skype is very functional, user-friendly, and most important, free. To download on your device, go to www.skype.com/en/. There is an easy-to-follow set of instructions on how to use Skype on the website.

Google Hangout

Developed in 2013 by Google, this telecommunication software is also free. Google Hangout allows for video conferencing with up to 10 users at the same time, making it a great option for community groups of birth professionals, birth networks, organizational boards of directors, or simply reaching a client when in-person meetings are not feasible. Should there be a need to hang out with 15 individuals at one time, a charge of less than $5 allows this option. Hangout chat histories can be saved for retrieving for note-taking.

Visit http://www.google.com/hangouts/ and take advantage of the instructional video.

Several more platforms, such as Sqwiggle and Facetime, will give Hangouts and Skype competition. While Sqwiggle is in its infancy at the time of publication, Facetime (an Apple product) can support (for free as long as all have the app downloaded) four people for a video chat, and nine people listening to audio only when used in combination with iChat / Messages. However, Facetime does not allow for screen sharing currently.

Regardless of which telecommunications software you choose to use, you will also need a dependable Internet connection. Picture freezing, or interruption in the voice communication, are common complaints of both Skype and Google Hangout. However, childbirth educators and doulas have been using Skype for years to connect families for birth services, including military family members not able to be available in-person for classes or births.

Worksheet 5

Social Media Marketing

Check Off	Business Goal	Social Media Option
	Establish yourself as an expert in your field with useful frequently updated information.	Create your website(s). Make this option colorful and dynamic!
	Continue to establish yourself as an expert with information in a more personal style.	Develop a blog, podcast, or even a YouTube video. Embed the video or podcast on the blog or website.
	Compile a community of networking: informational and with the potential of being customers.	Research Facebook, LinkedIn, and other social networks. Find one that best suits your needs.
	Give immediate updates to a specific group of people.	Twitter, Yahoo, or Instant Messaging
	Complete the circle of Social Media.	Link website to blog to Facebook to Twitter and close the circle!

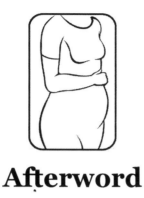

Afterword

Creating and Marketing Your Birth-Related Business is not a new topic to me. I have been presenting conference workshops in marketing for birth professionals since 1988, and incorporate small portions of this information in every professional training workshop I teach.

So many doulas and childbirth educators left workshops armed with the tools necessary to support their clients and teach classes, but had no clue how to turn their passion into a legal entity, protect their family, and become an established business in their community. Marketing has certainly changed since 1988, and with the help of the Internet (websites, blogs, Facebook, etc), a whole new avenue of marketing is before us. I feel blessed to have had the expertise of my daughter, too, to help me add so much to this topic.

Birth professionals are standing at the threshold of a new era in birth. Now all we have to do is push the door open.

I wish you all of the best in your endeavors.

~ Connie Livingston

References

Abarbanel, K., & Freeman, B. (2008). *Birthing the elephant: The woman's go-for-it! guide to overcoming the big challenges of launching a business.* Berkeley, CA: Ten Speed Press.

Brennan, P. (2014). *The doula business guide: Creating a successful mother-baby business,* 2nd edition. Ann Arbor, MI: Center for the Childbearing Year Press.

Brown, S. (2012). *How to create a successful holistic practice from start to succeed.* Amazon Digital.

Consumer Dummies. (2015). *Starting a business all-in-one for dummies.* Hoboken, NJ: Wiley.

Diamond, S. (2008). *Webmarketing for small businesses: 7 steps to explosive business growth.* Naperville, IL: Sourcebooks, Inc.

Fishman, S. (2012). *Deduct it! Lowering your small business taxes, 9th Edition.* San Francisco: NOLO.

Freeman, K. (2012). *How social media, mobile are playing a bigger part in healthcare.* Retrieved from: http://mashable.com/2012/12/18/social-media-mobile-healthcare/

Goldstein, B. (2007). *The ultimate small business marketing toolkit: All the tips, forms and strategies you'll ever need.* New York: McGraw-Hill.

Hawn, C. (2011). Take two aspirin and tweet me in the morning: How twitter, facebook, and other social media are reshaping health care. *Health Affairs, 28*(2) 361-368.

Health Research Institute. (2012). *Social media "likes" healthcare: From marketing to social business.* Retrieved from: www.download.pwc.com/ie/pubs/2012_social_media_likes_healthcare.pdf.

Hinmon, D. (2011). *Social media strategy blog.* Retrieved from: http://www.hivestrategies.com/2011/06/3-high-touch-ideas-to-inspire-your-hospital-social-media/

Kish-Doto, J. (2010). RUprego? The role of social media to educate young women about low-intervention childbirth. *Cases in Public Health Communication & Marketing, IV,* Summer, 3-7.

KMS Publishing. (2010). *Branding by blogging: Build your brand identity and online presence to the maximum sing this ultimate business branding strategy and the power of blogs.* North Charleston, SC: CreateSpace Independent Publishing Platform.

Larson, J. (2014). *New principles guide nurses in using social media*. Retrieved from: www.nursezone.com/printArticle.aspx?articleID=38004

Morris, T., & McInerney, K. (2010). Media representations of pregnancy and childbirth: An analysis of reality television programs in the United States. *Birth, 37*(2), 134-140.

Pakroo, P. (2014). *Small business startup kit*. San Francisco: NOLO Press.

Rain, A. (2013). *The ultimate "how to" guide for doulas: How to become a doula and create a successful business doing what you love*. Murray, UT: Infinite Rain Publishing.

Reuters News Service. (2010). Text messages save pregnant Rwandan women. Retrieved from: http//www.reuters.com/.

Romano, A., Gerber, H., & Andrews, D. (2010). Social media, power and the future of VBAC. *Journal of Perinatal Education, 19*(3), 43-52.

Schenck, B.F (2012). *Small business marketing for dummies, 3rd Edition*. San Francisco: Wiley Publishing.

Stelzner, M. (2007). *Writing white papers.* Retrieved from: http://www.writingwhitepapers.com/book/index.html

Tracy, B. (n.d.). *Get customers to sell for you.* Retrieved from: http://www.briantracy.com/blog/sales-success/get-customers-to-sell-for-you/

Tyson, E., & Schell, J. (2011). *Small business for dummies,* 4th Edition. San Francisco: Wiley Publishing.

Zak, P. J. (2008). The neurobiology of trust. *Scientific American.*

Zak, P. J. (2011). Trust, morality, and oxytocin. TED Talk.

Zak P. J., Stanton, A. A., & Ahmadi, S. (2007). Oxytocin increases generosity in humans. *PLoS ONE,* 2(11), e1128. doi:10.1371/journal

Internet References

https://business.pinterest.com/en

https://business.instagram.com/

http://www.entrepreneur.com/article/230488

http://www.squidoo.com/word-of-mouth-advertising

http://www.copyright.gov/help/faq/faq-general.html

http://psychology.about.com/od/sensationandperception/a/colorpsych.htm

http://www.eruptingmind.com/communication-gestures-vary-different-cultures/

http://www.asmp.org/tutorials/21st-century-worries.html

http://www.businessdictionary.com/definition/marketing.html

http://www.netmba.com/marketing/mix/

http://www.asmp.org/tutorials/property-and-model-releases.html

www.websourcellc.com

www.birthsource.com

http://www.icea.org/sites/default/files/Social%20Media%20HIPAA%20PP-FINAL.pdf

https://business.pinterest.com/en

https://business.instagram.com/

http://theundercoverrecruiter.com/8-steps-writing-bio-pro-chris-brogan-fact/

http://www.businessnewsdaily.com/7444-5-small-business-success-tips-for-women-entrepreneurs.html

http://www.webs.com/blog/2013/05/20/4-great-places-to-find-small-business-networking-events/

www.sba.gov

http://www.irs.gov/pub/irs-pdf/fw9.pdf

About the Authors

Connie Livingston, a birth researcher, journalist, and childbirth educator, founded Perinatal Education Associates, Inc. in 1999. A three-time March of Dimes "D.I.M.E." (Distinction in Media Excellence) award winner, and recognized by the Ohio House of Representatives for her work in maternity care, she also manages two websites, 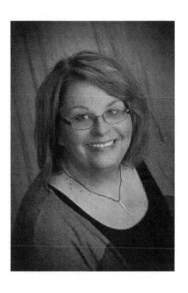 a blog, two Facebook pages, Pinterest and Instagram accounts, and she Tweets! Devoted to the dissemination of evidence-based maternity care, Connie is the author of over 1,300 published articles and three books. Her company has two websites: www.birthsource.com and www.thebirthfacts.com, a blog www.childbirthtoday.blogspot.com, and is present on Facebook, www. facebook.com/Birthsource, and Twitter, www.twitter. com/birthsourcecom.

Connie graduated with a degree in nursing in 1976 and sociology in 1978 from Purdue University. In 1997, she became Purdue University's first Outstanding Nursing Alumna Award recipient. She is a frequent speaker at birth conferences, and teaches doula and childbirth educator training workshops. In 2013, Connie became the International Childbirth Education Association (ICEA) President-Elect, and in 2015, assumed her role as President of ICEA. Connie lives in Dayton, Ohio with her husband, Jim. They have two daughters, Heather and Erin.

****

Heather Livingston is a proud Eastern Michigan University alumna. She obtained her Master's in Business Administration in 2004, as well as two bachelor degrees, one in International Business and the other French Language 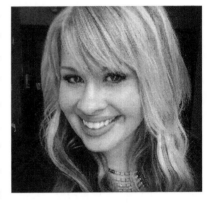 in 2002. She has worked in Higher Education for over 10 years, currently working for the University of Michigan as the Student Affairs Capital Projects Program Manager. For various offices and initiatives, she has developed marketing campaigns, social media outreach, websites, logos, newsletters, and printed marketing materials. She lives in Ann Arbor, Michigan.

Made in the USA
Middletown, DE
19 November 2019